OVERTHINKING DISORDER

How to Stop Worrying, Reduce Stress, Eliminate Negative Thinking

(Stop Negative Thinking, Good Habits and Much More)

Stephen Snyder

Published by Knowledge Icons

Stephen Snyder

Overthinking Disorder: How to Stop Worrying, Reduce Stress, Eliminate Negative Thinking (Stop Negative Thinking, Good Habits and Much More)

ISBN 978-1-990084-65-2

Legal & Disclaimer

The information contained in this book is not designed to replace or take the place of any form of medicine or professional medical advice. The information in this book has been provided for educational and entertainment purposes only.

The information contained in this book has been compiled from sources deemed reliable, and it is accurate to the best of the Author's knowledge; however, the Author cannot guarantee its accuracy and validity and cannot be held liable for any errors or omissions. Changes are periodically made to this book. You must consult your doctor or get professional medical advice before using any of the suggested remedies, techniques, or information in this book.

Upon using the information contained in this book, you agree to hold harmless the Author from and against any damages, costs, and expenses, including any legal fees potentially resulting from the application of any of the information provided by this guide. This disclaimer applies to any damages or injury caused by the use and application, whether directly or indirectly, of any advice or information presented, whether for breach of contract, tort, negligence, personal injury, criminal intent, or under any other cause of action.

You agree to accept all risks of using the information presented inside this book. You need to consult a professional medical practitioner in order to ensure you are both able and healthy enough to participate in this program.

Table of Contents

Introduction

Overthinking is very common and debilitating. It can hinder you from socializing, from having a sound sleep, affect your performance at work, and even disrupt a well-planned vacation. When overthinking becomes chronic, it can lead to both physical and mental discomfort. In summary, overthinking can leave you both physically and mentally exhausted. If this is how you feel at the moment, you might have attempted various ways of escaping from such a depressing situation with no success.

But then, what is overthinking disorder? Under normal circumstances, we all worry about one thing or another but when such anxieties begin to suck the life out of us, then it becomes a serious problem. Although not everyone will suffer from such degree of worries, some individuals are more prone to suffer from such disorders than others - especially people with a past record of anxiety disorder. Scientists have discovered that overthinking can activate various areas of the brain that regulate anxiety and fear.

But even if you never had a history of anxiety disorder, you might still be prone to overthinking, especially if you assume the responsibility of being a "problem-solver". Your greatest strength as an analytical thinker can end up becoming your greatest enemy, especially when you get stuck in a quagmire of unproductive thoughts. Also, feelings of uncertainty to a high degree can induce overthinking disorder. For instance, if a significant change such as a major loss occurred in your life, you might lose control of your mind and it may spin in an unproductive obsessiveness direction.

It is comforting to learn that one can overcome overthinking (and anxiety). There are many effective techniques for solving anxieties, no matter the cause, be it overthinking due to a failed relationship, health, or financial issues. Stay tuned, as this book takes you through the techniques of how to stop overthinking. But first, this book will start by defining each problem and then discussing the most effective solutions for each problem.

Human beings are hardwired for personal connections because our relationships complete us and fill the void. This is one reason we are always looking to form fruitful relationships. However, most of the time, the relationships we form becomes a burden. We are not able to sustain them or feel constrained by them. We start feeling the relationships to be a burden.

This inability to sustain relationships has become a widespread phenomenon for some time. It can lead to unhappiness, discontent, and mental fatigue.

It is important to understand that relationships are two-way connections. Unrealistic expectations in relationships contribute to the problems. It isn't the other partner in the relationship that causes the friction, but your expectation from the partner. If you are expecting something from your partner, you may become disappointed. Even setting rules doesn't help in this case as it is not a matter of receiving but perception.

Expectations from any relationship can cloud your thinking process. You come in the receiving mode and you start quantifying the unquantifiable. As a result, mutual trust and respect start fading. You become more and more demanding and less forgiving and accepting. Each and everything keeps getting registered in your mind and clutters it; the reactions arising in such cases are instinctive.

If you want to have healthy relationships, then being instinctive should be shunned. Mindfulness is the only way to cultivate nourishing relationships. You cannot let your mind clutter and prejudices rule your relationship. The clutter in your mind would make you unreceptive and unjustified. It will inflate your ego and make you unkind and uncompassionate.

Chapter 1: What Is Overthinking?

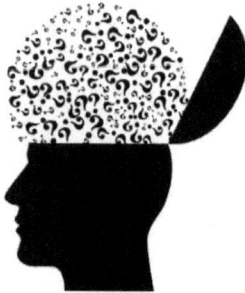

When you think excessively, rather than acting and getting things done, you are overthinking. When you examine, remark and rehash similar contemplations over and over rather than acting, you are overthinking.

This propensity keeps you from making a move. It devours your vitality, handicaps your capacity to decide, and puts you on a circle of thinking and thinking over and once more.

This is a sort of thinking that squanders your time and vitality and keeps you from acting, doing new things and gaining ground in your life. It resembles binds yourself to a rope that is associated with a post and going in circles over and over.

In this circumstance, there is a greater probability for stress, nervousness, and the absence of inward harmony. Then again, when you do not overthink, you become increasingly productive, progressively tranquil and increasingly upbeat.

What happens when you overthink? Well, you cannot quit thinking about an occasion, an individual, something that occurred before, or on an issue. Rather than searching for an answer, stepping up and being dynamic, you simply continue thinking and can't get it insane.

Now and again, when something awful occurs, you consider the most noticeably terrible situations, with musings like "imagine a scenario in which?" or "why. You slip once in a while into negative thinking designs.

You stress over past missteps or current issues and issues, and how they may prompt negative results. You fixate on or over-dissect your everyday encounters and collaborations with individuals. You blow up each word, thought and occasion past extremely and sensible extents, perusing into it things that aren't entirely.

On the off chance that this happens frequently, you are what clinicians call a ruminator or an over-scholar. Clinicians have discovered that over-thinking can be unfavorable to execution and lead to uneasiness and melancholy.

Uneasiness and overthinking will, in general, be malicious accomplices. One of the repulsive signs of a nervousness issue is the propensity to overthink everything. The brain is hyper-cautious, consistently watchful for anything it deems to be perilous or troubling. Overthinkers are often blamed for making issues where there are not any. However, there are, without a doubt, issues because anxiety makes anyone overthink everything. Tension makes us overthink everything from numerous points of view, and the aftereffect of this overthinking is not useful in any way. Luckily, tension and overthinking everything does not need to be a lasting piece of our reality.

What are the ways anxiety causes overthinking? Well, a significant impact of anxiety is overthinking everything. There are basic subjects to the manner in which tension causes overthinking. Maybe this conventional rundown will help you to remember explicit dashing contemplations you experience and help you understand that you are not the only one in overthinking everything as a result of tension.

Fixating on what we should say while being troubled with anxiety, agonizing perpetually over our identity and how we are measuring up to the world. This is actually normal in social situations.

Sometimes, making frightful imaginations about a scenario where situations about things that could turn out badly for ourselves, friends and family, and the world, regularly in summed up anxious situations.

Wild, envisioned aftereffects of our own wild, envisioned deficiencies and inadequacies, the dread of having a fit of anxiety in broad daylight and potentially thinking that you cannot leave home as a result of it.

Agonizing over a large number of fanatical considerations, some of the time alarming ones and thinking about them continually causes you to think too much. Overthinking, a tumbling chain of stresses, unclear contemplations, and explicit considerations.

With anxiety, not exclusively are these considerations going through our minds, yet they are continually going through our cerebrums, constant, unendingly. Like a gerbil snared to an unending trickle of a caffeinated drink, they run and run and wheel around in one spot, going completely no place. Day and night, the wheel squeaks.

Over-thinking everything is an appalling anxious situation. Over-thinking everything creates more tension within you. This tip helps to stop over-thinking. Anxiety and overthinking everything makes us both worn out and wired. One consequence of thinking in excess is that we are frequently left physically and genuinely unwell. Having these equivalent restless messages gone through our mind wherever we go causes significant damage.

Further, another perilous consequence of nervousness and overthinking everything is that we begin to accept what we think. All things considered, on the off chance that we think it, it is genuine, and if we think it continually, it is genuine. This is a trap where nervousness plays. Uneasiness causes overthinking, yet with nervousness, these contemplations are not constantly reliable.

You have the power and the capacity to overcome anxiety and overthinking everything. It is a procedure that includes numerous means, however, a stage you can bring right presently to hinder that gerbil is to have something with you or around you to occupy your consideration. Instead of contending with your considerations or fixating on them, delicately move your consideration onto something different, something nonpartisan. By thinking about something inconsequential, you weaken the capacity of anxiety to make you overthink everything.

Chapter 2: Signs You Are An Overthinker

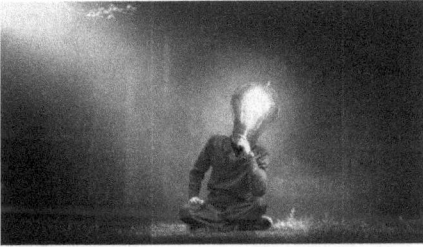

Chronic fatigue. The brain is at its maximum capacity when overthinking takes hold of your attention. Since the brain is a power-hungry organ system, it consumes a great deal of your usual energy. Hence, you may find yourself constantly tired bordering on exhaustion. This is why you often need more sleep than most folks.

Overanalyzing everything. The chronic overthinkers make something out of everything. Even when someone makes a very innocent comment, the overthinker will find something and blow it out of proportion. Often, it is just a ploy to get the attention they crave.

Dread of disappointment. The knit-picking tendencies of the overthinker lead them to constant disappointment. Since it is virtually impossible for them to take anything at face value, they will try to find the catch in everything. This leads to constant disappointment.

Failure to be in the now. The overthinker is generally concerned about the past and focused on the future. This leads them to forget about living in the present, that is, enjoying life's most precious moments, and the people around them.

Continually re-thinking themselves. In other words, the overthinker is constantly second-guessing themselves, making unreasonable criticisms about themselves and the things they have done or failed to.

Constant headaches. Given the fact that the brain is at full blast, the overthinker is generally prone to headaches. It is only when these folks are able to calm down that they find peace and solace in the world around them.

Chronic sleeping disorders. Since overthinkers are prone to insomnia, they tend to be sleep deprived until their bodies shut down. At that point, they may oversleep as the body attempts to recoup precious rest.

Stiff muscles and joints. A chronic overthinker is in a constant state of stress. This may lead to maintain a consistent state of stiffness in joints and muscles. Hence, aches and pains throughout the body are very common.

Living in dread. There is the overwhelming sensation of impending doom no matter how cut and dry things may be. After all, there is always the possibility that something could go wrong regardless of how far-fetched it may be.

If you can relate to these characteristics, then it would be a great idea to find a person in whom you can trust, who can listen to you, so that you can ventilate at least some of your feelings as often as you can.

Chapter 3: Anxiety And Overthinking

Probably someone has once accused you of always creating problems for yourself out of insignificant issues. Personally, I think they are actually problems. How so? Simply put, anxiety makes you overthink anything and everything. Whenever we are anxious, we overthink things in various ways, and the product of our overthinking is not often beneficial. However, anxiety and overthinking should be temporary and should not be a permanent feature of our existence.

Ways anxiety causes overthinking

The end product of various types of anxiety is overthinking everything. There are various terms to describe how anxiety leads to overthinking. It is possible that this generic list will help you recall specific racing thoughts which you may have experienced or are likely experiencing and thus, help you realize that there are thousands of other individuals facing the same problem.

Being overly concerned about who we are and how others view us or if we are measuring up to the world standard (this is a form of social and performance anxiety).

Obsessing over what we should say/said/should have said/shouldn't say (another common social anxiety).

Thinking about fearful possible scenarios such as: what if something bad should happen to us, our loved ones, or even the world (a common form of generalized anxiety disorder).

Fearful, assumed results of our own wild thoughts, assumed faults, and feelings of incompetence (all forms of anxiety disorders).

Anxiety over multiple obsessive thoughts, mostly scary ones, and thinking about them continually (a form of obsessive, compulsive disorder).

Thinking, overthinking, vague thoughts, a tumbling chain of anxiety, and specific thoughts (all forms of anxiety disorders).

Fear of experiencing panic attacks in public and feeling too scared to leave home due to such anxiety (a form of panic disorder with/without agoraphobia).

Result of anxiety and overthinking

When you're anxious, the thoughts do not just run through your brain and disappear, rather, they run through your brain continuously. Those thoughts can be compared to an athlete running on a treadmill, he keeps running but gets nowhere in the end, left wired and tired. One of the side effects of overthinking linked with anxiety is that we are likely to end up both physically and emotionally drained. Having bouts of the same anxious impulses run through our brain will definitely take its toll.

Another dark side of anxiety and overthinking is that sooner or later, we will begin to perceive everything that goes through our mind as reality. Perhaps we may believe that what we think about becomes reality and if we constantly think about it, it becomes very real. Right? No. This is one of the tricks anxieties tries to play on our minds.

But the good news is, we all have the capacity and the power to stop ourselves from being anxious and overthinking everything. Although, this is a process that involves multiple steps, at the moment, the best step you can take is to find something that can distract you from overthinking. Instead of battling with your thoughts, lowly divert your attention to something neutral, something else entirely. By pondering over something that is of no significance, you will be indirectly preventing overthinking everything.

The "leaven" effect

Overthinking has a "leaven effect" on your thoughts. Just like a dough, your mind can knead negative thoughts and, before you know it, it will rise to twice the initial size.

For instance, if a customer is dissatisfied with your services, you may begin to wonder if all the other customers are dissatisfied as well without giving it a second thought that probably most of the customers might actually be satisfied with your services. If care is not taken, with time, you might come to a discouraging conclusion that your services are not good enough. Your thoughts can even take you back to your marriage and you might begin to wonder if your mate is satisfied with you or if you're good enough for her or not. You think about how perfect she is, how she handles everything impressively, and conclude that you're totally unworthy of her.

The "distorted lens" effect

Another effect of overthinking is what is called the "distorted lens" effect and what this means, is that your thoughts only focus and magnify your faults or bad side and what your thoughts see is only hopelessness. For instance, when your kid comes home from school with a poor grade or gets into a fight, you may worry that he or she is growing up badly. Before long, you will start seeing yourself as a bad parent and that later in the future, your children will end up becoming bad adults.

What Overthinking Is Not

Worrying is quite different from overthinking. People often worry about things that can or may happen or possibly go wrong. Overthinkers; however, do more than just worry about the present, they also worry about the past and the future as well. While worriers think that bad things might happen; over thinkers think backward and they are very convinced that something bad had already happened.

Individuals with obsessive-compulsive disorder (OCD) are also different from overthinking. Those with OCD are overly obsessed about everything or every external factor, such as dirt or germs so they feel they have to wash their hands repeatedly to stay healthy. Such ones obsess about very specific actions and other matters that appear trivial or absurd to the rest of the world, such as "Did I lock the door?"

Chapter 4: What Is Negativity?

Now In life, there are always two sides to a phenomenon. Here there is positivity, and there is negativity. Have you ever just bumped into some really angry, grumpy, and frustrated people who will just hurl words at you for nothing, and find every viable opportunity to give off their bad vibe? Well I've not implied that they are negative people, but I guess you already did. Yes, your face says it all.

That was on a light note. But really, I think somewhere deep down in my heart that those people should undoubtedly equal as negatively minded people.

Navigating these scenarios of negativity well depends on your ability to be mindful of your thoughts and actions.

Negative Mindset

A negative mindset is one that rarely sees good in people, events or situations. They are the kind of people who would always have complaints to register, and excuses to make. They never see a thing or an idea going well. The moment you share an initiative with them, they'll be the first to make a list of a hundred and one reason why it wont work, and they won't stop at that. They'll help you ridicule your convictions to the point where you'll begin to believe that they are right.

Watch out for negative minded people. Another tool they use is blame. They are never responsible for the failure of anything committed to their hands. Well, they might be right because chances are that they had already informed the supervisor of the task that it will not work, right from the start. Whether a negative or positive mindset, the underlying factor that differentiates them both is focus. Whatever it is that you concentrate more on will determine your mindset. A positive minded person will always see hope, a way out, and a future in whatever is committed to him. But those that utter words like:

It's just impossible

We can't

It is too complex

We are not enough

It cannot work

And other words that share same worldview with these phrases are negative minded. These words are such that will continually characterise the speech of a negative minded person.

The next time you find yourself uttering these words too often, or making incessant blame on yourself, others, the circumstances, or the universe for whatever is happening to you, then you should watch it.

And in the event that you notice some negative trends, although it may sound rather dire, but remember that there is a solution for negative thinking, and it is very much within your reach.

How Does Negativity Influence Us?

Most negative people often say they are the happiest because they have set themselves in positions where disappointment cannot reach. But in reality, negativity makes people feel sad, hopeless and grumpy. It just leaves them living life as someone who is unexpectant of anything. And anyone who is unexpectant only just waits for time to drag by without anything happy or exciting ever happening. We should understand that Negativity not only affects our emotions and thinking behavior, but it hurts the ones we love, and reduces them to little piece of tools to us.

You know the funny thing? The funny thing about this phenomenon that we all are castigating is the fact that nobody is immune to it. To put it lightly everyone catches the negativity syndrome every once in a while. But the difference is that while some people make efforts at fighting it when it comes, some people just wallow in it, allowing their emotions to control them. And another sect of people consciously and deliberately make negativity their life pattern and habit.

I'm sure that is why you have this book in your hand at such a time as this. Because you sure fall into the category of one of the earlier mentioned sects. So, together, let's take that step into positivity and away from negativity. It'll be an honor to help you through this journey.

Chapter 5: Optimizing Relief From Stress

And Anxiety

Sooner or later in time, everybody encounters pressure and anxiety in their life. Be that as it may, a few people will in general be more pressure solid than others, and can all the more effectively adapt to the horrendous emotions and physical responses that pressure and anxiety cause. A ton of books, articles, and studies have been composed and directed about how to beat pressure. I'm going to include one more thought I've observed to be valuable from my examination, and after that portray why I think it works so well.

A typical strategy utilized to conquer pressure is to contemplate. For what reason would contemplation be compelling? A large number of the logical reports make no cases as to comprehend the thinking other than to note contemplation can bring down one's pulse and moderate one's mind wave capacities. In spite of the fact that I can't guarantee medicinal or explore certifications behind my name, I'll try the clarification of why contemplation works by looking at the profound cover with the physical action. As it were, so as to comprehend why reflection works, we have to inspect the mechanics of the occasion to perceive what's going on.

A reflection session may begin with the announcement of an issue and a solicitation for direction and understanding. At that point, when an individual ponders, she eases back her psyche to the point where she attempts to consider nothing by any stretch of the imagination. This is the place that enchantment occurs. At the point when the brain is calmed, an extension is basically unblocked between one's cognizant and intuitive personalities. The subliminal personality has a higher-level point of view on the occasions that are happening in one's life, and can give knowledge - and conceivably even replies to a significant number of life's inquiries and issues. The alleged "hard" part is just setting aside a few minutes throughout your life to calm your brain and enable that association to happen. By introducing the issues or occasions that are causing us to worry to our higher awareness to understand, we utilize a higher and more astute point of view from which we can figure out how to conquer our issues. Frequently we locate a degree of acknowledgment or comprehension through this undertaking that can enable us to discover brief and even supportable alleviation from the negative effects of pressure and anxiety.

I'd like to include one more thought that I have observed to be episodically compelling at battling pressure and anxiety in my own life. It likely could be that the disturbing occasions we involvement in life were structured by us (for example our oversoul) before we were ever conceived, and are intended to move us to discover an answer or defeat some difficulty. In the event that this is valid, at that point the best way to move past that preliminary is to acknowledge it, maybe even offer gratitude for it(!), and afterward request the direction and solidarity to survive and move past this preliminary. You can do this through a quiet and gathering petition, just as reflection; whichever is most agreeable for you. It might sound odd to "acknowledge" or even "offer gratitude" for a preliminary in life that has caused an untold measure of agony and enduring, yet in the event that you can comprehend the preliminary from a higher perspective for example as a major aspect of one's required beneficial experience then you are one bit nearer to conquering that hardship in record time. This is likewise, I dare say, an indication of an individual who is astoundingly pressured strong as they can acknowledge and beat distressing occasions in their existence with insignificant trouble. But then, we see from these discoveries that conquering pressure and anxiety, and getting to be pressure tough is a range of abilities that anybody can learn.

HOW TO OVERCOME STRESS AND ANXIETY TO PREVENT DEPRESSION

Stress is a characteristic reaction of our body to considered dangers and weights throughout everyday life; while anxiety is essentially an inclination of stress, anxiety, or an extraordinary misgiving of genuine or envisioned risk. It could likewise be a solid wish to accomplish something, particularly if the desire is unfortunate solid; like being on edge to make the best decision. Hence, anxiety may now and again happen because of an absence of trust in self.

Both stress and anxiety are typical responses in our bodies because of difficult circumstances throughout everyday life. They are impermanent occasions that vanish once those apparent dangers and weights are no more. In any case, should they remain longer than typical, at that point it relapsed to some type of despondency.

How to Overcome Stress and Anxiety to Prevent Depression? Give us an initial chance to comprehend the reason why you have this sentiment of stress and anxiety? Anxiety is a side effect of the nearness of uncertainty, and when there is a question, fear grasps in. At the point when fear grasps in, anxiety comes in. All these; uncertainty, fear, and anxiety are appearances of a negative mental frame of mind, drawing in progressively negative things to occur. The more extraordinary the anxiety, the more what you feared of, will prone to occur. Why? In view of the Law of Attraction; the more you contemplate it, the more you will get it.

So the best thing to beat anxiety is to defeat your negative mental frame of mind. Have you seen that when there is something that you don't care to occur, it's bound to occur? A case of this is the point at which you were in school when the instructor calls haphazardly for someone to display before the class; you would prefer not to exhibit since you are not readied, or you are not certain to show; what do you feel? You felt on edge, on edge that you may be called. The more restless you become, the more probable that you will be called. Also, in the event that you were restless, at that point certainly, you were called.

In the Law of Attraction, the procedure begins with having an idea of what you need; at that point, this idea changes to have what you need. Want is a feeling, amazing enough to lead you to activity until you get what you what. Anxiety is as of now a feeling, an amazing inclination that will lead you to your overwhelming negative idea that something you feared of.

How at that point do you defeat your negative mental frame of mind? To defeat a negative mental disposition is to have a positive mental frame of mind. You can not defeat a negative mental frame of mind with a negative mental demeanor. Give me a chance to give you a model: As I perused the Google catchphrase, I saw that many individuals looked through Google about anxiety, around 4 million inquiries in a single month, contrasted with satisfaction at around a million of each month. Both of these gatherings of individuals who scanned for anxiety and joy are bound to experience the ill effects of anxiety or discouragement. In the event that you are cheerful, for what reason would you look for joy on the web at any rate? The distinction between these gatherings of individuals is their methodology or how they dealt with their anxiety. Four million attempted to deal with their anxiety by becoming familiar with anxiety. They wind up nourishing their contemplations increasingly about anxiety, accounts of individuals with anxiety, etc. They wind up pulling in increasingly negative powers to them and become progressively on edge. Then again, those individuals who attempted to fight their anxiety by developing their musings with upbeat considerations, glad minutes, tales about bliss; and encircle themselves with cheerful individuals are bound to prevail in regards to defeating their anxiety.

Stress and anxiety are mental perspectives where negative musings are overwhelming, making questions and fears. To beat stress and anxiety is to pick up authority over your contemplations and to change your psychological demeanor to an inspirational attitude. What's more, perhaps the most ideal approach to have a constructive mental frame of mind is to sustain your psyche with glad contemplations, vivacious music, cheerful minutes, and partner yourself with upbeat individuals.

LEARN THE NATURAL WAYS TO RELEASE STRESS AND ANXIETY FAST

Living is great, despite the fact that life can be testing. For some people, only the idea of confronting the world and intermingling with others can be somewhat troublesome. For a few, it can even be excruciating, but then there are as yet the individuals who can't carry themselves ever to confront the present reality as they become hermetic. A significant number of these people will experience the ill effects of the impacts of low self-certainty until they find out about the regular approaches to discharge stress and anxiety.

Youth Traumas and Influences of Others

A few people endure the stress of youth injuries and the impacts of others. This will expand the odds of certain people to encounter troubles when attempting to cooperate with others whether they are relatives, companions, work partners, or managers in sentimental connections. Pressures can develop that may cause different issues or the compounding of existing issues for the individual and the people around them.

On the off chance that any person who is experiencing the staggering emotions and musings of melancholy does not find a way to improve their personal satisfaction, they need to keep enduring pointlessly. It isn't so natural to discharge stress when you don't have the slightest idea of how to do so. In any case, there are many fascinating ways that you can conquer stress and anxiety.

Looking for Answers

Looking for answers that are useful and clever is one of the initial steps to helping yourself feel good. Remember that you are not the only one and you don't need to endure this alone. There is help for you, and there are numerous things you can accomplish for yourself to beat the difficulties you're confronting.

Battling Negative Thinking

Negative reasoning will impact the manner in which you consider things, the manner in which you talk and feel about different issues. The thing about negative reasoning is that in the event that you don't play a functioning job in battling it, it can demolish your life. Along these lines, it just bodes well that anybody experiencing the impact of negative reasoning will recognize it, and after that work towards making an improvement. You can improve the manner in which you think and feel by utilizing uplifting feedback and positive reasoning and confirmations.

Exploit accessible Resources

When you are looking for assistance, you can discover countless accessible assets on the web. For example, there are numerous useful sites and web journals that offer incredible data about figuring out how to unwind. You can learn a wide range of elective methods that will enable you to conquer stress, anxiety and melancholy. You may likewise discover numerous supportive eBooks that give you valuable data. Take a stab at learning distinctive exercise schedules until you discover one that is agreeable for you and helps to discharge stress. Set aside the effort to look online and to discover supportive assets.

Change your Thinking and Change your Life

On the off chance that you are enduring and you ceaselessly intimidated yourself, you are not doing whatever can enable you to improve life. Be that as it may, on the off chance that you figure out how to change your reasoning, you can transform you.

Take the time presently to become familiar with the various strategies that can enable you to feel solid improvement. You can gain proficiency with the normal approaches to discharge stress and anxiety in a quick and incredible nature. Do it today.

Chapter 6: Rewire Your Brain For

Positivity

It is natural and normal to think negative thoughts because your brain automatically generates them. However, you do have the power to change the way your mind works and reset your default way of thinking to positive.

Automatic negative thoughts can be overwhelming and make you feel anxious and depressed. They are not pleasant, but you can deal with them and change the narrative.

How you deal with negative thoughts

You need to realize that they are

•Not true

•Unhelpful

•Designed to keep you from moving on

•The key reason you feel anxious or depressed

Automatic negative thoughts

"Always trust your feelings" is fine for some people but when your first response is a negative one does this mean you should believe it? No, it doesn't. Recognizing this fact can change your life and your thinking. Consider the following phrases and if you automatically think like this then you need to rewire your thoughts:

Someone gives you a compliment about your appearance and you think: "They don't mean it" or "They must be lying"

Something great happens to you and you hear this phrase in your head; "Why me, I don't deserve this" or "Something will happen to take this away from me"

You meet a group of strangers and you think: "They will all hate me and wonder why I am here" or "Nobody wants to meet me, I'm not good company"

You need to challenge these thoughts and recognize that automatic responses are not truthful. You must stop them from running your life and making you miserable. The next time you have a negative thought ask yourself one simple question, "How true is this thought?" and then analyze the answer.

For instance, take the phrase "nobody likes me" that can often crop up in our thoughts. Replace this with a deliberate thought such as "ok, have I met everybody in the world, the country or even my town? No, I haven't, neither has there been a survey done on my likeability so how can I think nobody likes me?" Doing so allows you to distinguish between what you believe and what you know. This is a positive way to think and helps you dispel the automatic negativity in your mind.

There are multiple ways to deal with them and these two examples could be the ones for you:

1) Imagine the thoughts are outside your head: This technique allows you to manage the thoughts and decide what to do with them. Once any negativity begins to form just refuse to let it in. State clearly

and with conviction "No, I refuse to allow negative thoughts to enter my head". Repeat the word "no" until the thoughts disappear.

2)   If you find it difficult to dispel the thoughts try adding words to them to change the narrative. For instance, if your thought is "I hate my job and I am terrible at it" add positive elements to form "I hate my job so I am going to look for another, I know that I am good at….." Another way to change perspective can be "Life is pointless" will become "Life is pointless if you don't make the most of it".

Negative thoughts often occur at regular times of the day or are triggered by certain locations. Knowing what triggers your negative thought process can help you be more alert and ready to deal with them.

Programming your brain to be positive

Now we understand what negative thinking is and how to deal with it we have taken the first step to rewire the brain. The following exercises will expand on the process and allow the brain to be happy and recognize success. We can also overcome bad habits and make it easier to improve life in general.

Follow these tips to rewire your mind for positivity

1)   Recognize that you view positive and negative thoughts simultaneously: George Orwell created a term in his groundbreaking novel, 1984, called doublethink and described it as the process of holding two opposing thoughts in one's mind and giving them both the same consideration and acceptance simultaneously.

Doublethink describes perfectly the way your brain works when considering positive and negative thoughts. It values both and uses them to fit the situation. For instance, your brain can create thoughts that indicate a positive attitude to yourself. "I am a valuable member of society" and "I have no qualities to offer the world" are two opposite opinions but can be given the same value in your head.

Rewiring your brain means you place less value on negative thoughts and automatically favor positive thoughts instead.

2) Identify your goals: Despite the phrase "seeing is believing" when setting goals in life we first must believe in them before we see results. Examine your goals and how they will manifest in your life. Believe that you will achieve them and imagine how your life will be when you have all you wish for.

3) Embrace positive emotions: Emotions are the fuel of the mind; they power our minds and bodies to strive for greater things and better intentions. Positive affirmations are only helpful if they stir the emotions and fire up the spirit. What emotions do you associate with accomplishments? Pride, happiness, elation or joy are all emotions we love to embrace. Recognize what your goals mean

to you and imagine the surge of emotion you will feel when you achieve them.

4)   Visualize: Your brain is the starting point for forming new habits. If you visualize images that accompany your goal, then your mind automatically increases your ability to create them in life. If you are committed to a future that is positive and fulfilling the images you create in your mind should reflect this. You will then begin to shape your actions to create a positive outcome you desire.

5)   Make your actions reflect your intentions: It is one thing to imagine positive actions but unless you actually make changes to your routine it will just be hot air! For instance, if your affirmations are all about eating healthier and getting yourself fit there is no point sitting down and eating burgers every day. There is also no point going to the gym but complaining about it. Rewiring your brain means embracing your new goals and

experiencing positive emotions as you do so.

Of course, this process requires commitment and practice. You have a lifetime of overthinking and negativity to overcome. Think of it in the same way you train a puppy: you need to catch it pooping on the carpet to house train it. This is how you rewire your brain; you catch it in the act of forming a negative thought and change the process.

Chapter 7: Learning To Reduce Stress And

Focus On Core Values

Evaluate Your Working and Living Environment

Whether at work or at home, your environment affects the way you feel and function. You need to do everything you can to make it a space in which you feel comfortable.

Now let's put our overcoming objections exercise to work.

Office 101: Is your workspace clear? Is it clean? Do you have a place for everything and is everything in that place? If you cannot answer yes to those three, then you have your place to start.

Stressed You: I have to work at work. I don't have time to be a maid or my own assistant. I work from the time I get there until I leave, **I don't waste time fooling around**.

Happy You: I think I see the problem. You seem to think that straightening up your workspace is a frivolous waste of time. But what about all that time you spend trying to find the scissors, staple remover, meeting agenda, or your buried glasses?

Solution: Happy You got it in one. Bite the bullet and try it for three weeks. Take the time after each project, task, or whatever you are working on and put everything back where it belongs. If it doesn't have a place, find one for it. Clear your desk; straighten your selves and draws.

Office 201: You don't have a problem with clutter or organization, but the atmosphere is drab and depressing. You really only have three choices.

Approach the powers that be about renovating or at least refreshing.

See what you can do to create a space in which you are comfortable. Plants, family pics, and mementos can help.

Look for a new job.

On the Home Front

If you don't get stuck at home and have a reasonably clean and organized house, then there is no need to ramp it up to the next level and go all Martha Stewart in every room. If you have clear, comfortable spaces for working, resting, and entertaining. No need to spend time in this area.

~ Don't own so much clutter that you will be relieved to see your house catch fire. ~
- Wendell Berry, Farming: a handbook

Singles with a Clutter Issue

If you have clutter issues or a stacking situation, then I'm guessing that you have been trying to get your house or apartment clean and clear for a while. **Think back, was there some incident that happened before items began accumulating?** If so, you might want some counseling help to resolve that particular issue. If you've always had a problem where you get shut down before you really get going with the clear out, what happens? Does a loop start in your head? Try the exercises from Chapter 2.

The one thing you never want to do is say: **"I'm not working on another project until this house is clean."** Because you never will work on another project. Start making new daily habits.

You need to work cleaning and clearing into your schedule. Get four empty boxes and set them out in front of you and grab your pad and pen. The box to your left is "keep and store" and you will need to write down where exactly you are going to put that item. The box directly in front of you is "Give Away" and the boxes to your right are "throwaway" and "recycle".

Pull one of your boxes or stacks and start. If you are keeping an item that you pull from your stack, write down an item description and exactly where you are going to put this item. You can do this while watching TV or listening to some of your favorite music.

When you have finished that first stack takes the "throwaway" and "recycle" box out and fill the bins. **That should feel amazing**. You just made room in your house to breathe and fill with love and positive energy. Now take the "Give Away" box and put that in your car to drop off at a suitable charity such as Goodwill or Salvation Army **tomorrow**. For the last box, the "keep and store" box, take the items and put them where they belong - **right now!**

~ If you missed your chance to read a particular book, even if it was recommended to you or is one you have been intending to read for ages, this is your chance to let it go. You may have wanted to read it when you bought it, but if you haven't read it by now, the book's purpose was to teach you that you didn't need it. There is no need to finish reading books that you only got halfway through. Their purpose was to be read halfway. So, get rid of all those unread books. It will be far better for you to read the book that really grabs you right now than one that you left to gather dust for years. ~

- Marie Kondo, The Life-Changing Magic of Tidying Up: The Japanese Art of Decluttering and Organizing

Families with a Clutter Issue

If you have family members call a meeting every two to three weeks and work, one new habit into each person's schedule.

Keeping Your Space Clean		
Name	**Date**	New Habit
Mom	2-May	Swiffer hard floors downstairs between vacuums
Dad	2-May	Leave work/yard boots on porch stand - use house shoes
Child 1	2-May	Wash sink each night
Child 2	2-May	Put clothes in hamper before bed

Mom	23-May	Don't let mail stack up - dispatch once a week
Dad	23-May	Help fold and distribute laundry
Child 1	23-May	Put away sports gear
Both kids	23-May	Bring used towels and bedsheets to laundry on Saturdays
Child 2	23-May	Put away your games, toys, and books after use.
		add as needed

What is Your Fuel?

~ It is easier to change a man's religion than to change his diet. ~

- Margaret Mead

You can't solve anything if you aren't taking care of yourself. If you have a diet, and by diet, I mean eating regimen, that keeps you fit and trim, wonderful. You may not need this segment, but I bet you know someone who might benefit from a new look at calorie consumption.

I'm going to talk about **macros** for a moment; they aren't just for bodybuilders anymore. Most of the diets you read about these days such as Paleo, Atkins, Keto, and others are formulated around increasing or decreasing the intake of carbohydrates, proteins, and fats.

Looking at food in terms of macros breaks down what is contained in the product so you can tell where your calories are coming from in the dish. Sounds complicated, but it really isn't. The percentages are conveniently contained on the product's nutrition label. For whole foods such as apple or cheddar cheese, there are online nutrient calculators that you can use to figure the percentage spread.

Below is what a typical day might look for a woman who would like to lose weight at a moderate rate.

		Portion	gCarbs	gProt	gFat	cCarbs	cProt	cFat	Calories
Br	Basted Egg with Smoked Salmon on Toast	1	28	13	19	112	52	171	335
Sn	Protein Drink	1	4	20	2	16	80	18	114
Ln	Shrimp Salad	1	16	30	15	64	120	135	319
S	Prot	1	12	2	4	48	8	3	92

n	...ein granola bar	Bar						6	
D n	Spicy Pan-Seared Salmon	6 oz.	0	33	17	0	132	153	285
	Steamed Asparagus	8 stalks	3	2	1	12	8	9	29
	Side Salad	small	3	1	0.5	12	4	4.5	20.5
S n	1/4 almonds, 1		6	12	21	24	48	189	261

	oz. cheese							
	Totals		72	113	80	288	452	716	1455.5

Carbohydrates, proteins, and **fats** are the three major nutrients contained in the food we eat. **They are called Macronutrients** or Macros for short.

A Quick Refresher Course

A reminder of what simple and complex **carbohydrates** are.

Simple carbs break down fast and are absorbed quickly into the bloodstream. Some foods considered simple carbs are: **refined sugar, fruit juice, candy, honey, white potatoes, white rice, refined white flour, alcohol, syrups, and sodas.**

Complex carbs, on the other hand, are released slowly in the bloodstream over a period of time to help sustain your body's energy. Some foods considered complex carbs are: quinoa, brown rice, beans, lentils, oatmeal, and peas.

Protein is not stored in the body but is found in almost every part of the body, nails, hair, skin, bone, muscle and tissue.

Fat is a bit more complicated. There is saturated fat such as lard or tallow (pork and beef fat), dairy fats, and some tropical oils (palm, palm kernel, and coconut). You want to keep your intake of these fats as low as possible

Trans fats are basically man-made fats created by hydrogenating oils (Crisco, commercial peanut butter). Check the label for trans-fat content or partially hydrogenated oil (code for trans-fat), and steer clear of these products.

Then there are the unsaturated fats:

Monounsaturated fats - olives, nuts, avocado, and seeds. Oils such as peanut, canola and olive oils.

Polyunsaturated fats: Omega-3 fatty acids can be found in walnuts, ground flaxseed, tofu and soybeans, canola, soybean and walnut oils. Many of the oily fish such as bluefish, herring, lake trout, mackerel, salmon, sardines, and tuna contain omega-3 fatty acids.

Omega-6 fatty acids sunflower seeds, Brazil nuts, pecans, and pine nuts. Cooking oils include corn, sunflower, safflower and sesame oils.

What is the difference between counting calories and counting macros?

When we count calories, we are counting the number of calories (energy) we consume from the food regardless of the nutrient source. When counting macros, we count the calories consumed from each of the nutrients.

This is the calculation you need to remember in order to find out where your calories come:

One gram of carbs = 4 calories

One gram of protein = 4 calories

One gram of fat = 9 calories

The basic ratio your body needs per day is 30% carbs, 40% protein, and 30% fat. Now, this can change depending on your personal health goals that you have set up with your physician.

Sex: M
Age: 35
Weight: 185
Height: 5' 11"
Exercise: 3 times a week, 30 minutes
Job: Sedentary
Maintain: 2472 calories
Moderate Fat Loss: 1978 calories
Extreme Fat Loss: 1483 calories
Sex: F
Age: 35
Weight: 170
Height: 5' 4"
Exercise: 3 times a week, 30 minutes
Job: Sedentary
Maintain: 2091 calories
Moderate Fat Loss: 1683 calories
Extreme Fat Loss: 1480 calories

There are many excellent sources of information for macro meal planning on the web. Team up this method of tracking calories with the Mediterranean diet and it's fairly painless to stick with the regimen. Your physician can get you started in the right direction.

A couple of tips for making a change in eating habits easier:

Keep a protein drink ready in the refrigerator so you can have a quick 20-gram protein pick up at a moment's notice instead of an entire meal.

Keep boiled eggs available, they are good on side salads and for a stand-alone snack.

Fish such as salmon, grouper, and snapper are an excellent source of low-fat protein.

Quinoa is a versatile source of complex carbohydrate that is good anything from breakfast dishes to chocolate bar snacks. It's not just good for a savory side.

Self-Medicating

Are you using drugs or alcohol to smooth out the rough edges? Does it make going to social outings easier? Or maybe it makes you feel better when certain memories pop up out of nowhere.

To figure out what your triggers are for self-medicating, flip back to the page that has your emotional triggers listed from chapter 2. Whatever form your self-medication takes, think about what set you off. Were you criticized or did you feel verbally attacked? Was it stress over money or a job? Lack of love or stuck in a bad relationship? What were you feeling? Angry, sad, out of control (fear), or guilt?

Make a note under the feeling or feelings that trigger the self-medicating. Put it right there in ink so that you can begin to heal and feel better.

~ A bear, however hard he tries, grows tubby without exercise. ~

- A.A. Milne, Winnie-the-Pooh

Get Moving

If you only choose one thing to implement per week, start with walking. You can do yourself a great benefit in both body and mind with a quick, brisk walk around the block. If you have not been exercising at all and are seriously out of shape, please check with your physician. If you do not have access to health care, start slow. A five to ten-minute walks to start, and then add a few minutes each week. In no time, you will be up to 30 minutes a day.

Not into Gyms

You don't have to join a gym and go all boot camp (there's that all or nothing mentality kicking in). Work more footsteps into your day. Park further away from the store or office. Ride a bike or take a bus to work. Take the stairs instead of using the elevator or escalator.

Many local parks now have Parcours courses. This is usually a jogging trail with a series of workout stations equipped with instructions on how to do the exercise. Go at your own pace and follow the trail around from station to station. Skip the ones that feel uncomfortable or cannot be accomplished at this time.

Wear a pedometer and make it a game to see if you can get to 10,000 steps each day. You would be surprised at some of the activities that really add up the steps. House cleaning and yard work are great ways to get the number of steps up.

Social Butterflies

If you want some company, check out your city's recreation department. They sometimes have some wonderful exercise classes at very reasonable rates. Dancing is a great way to lose weight while having fun. Zumba, Jazzercise, Belly Dancing, Ballroom Dancing, Country, Swing, Pole, Salsa, Hip-hop, and Clogging to name a few. Some require partners, some don't. Most have beginner introductory lessons that are meant to give you an idea of what you'll be doing in the class. Some are more strenuous than others, so you have a variety of fitness levels.

If you are fortunate enough to live near a university, college, or two-year college call them and see if they have any health science classes running for adults. These can be a great way to get back in shape with safe, experienced supervision. The trainers are often the staff and students who are highly trained professionals (or training to become professional in sports science). They can help tailor a workout that fits your time and skill level. You will also learn more about how your body works and what it needs to live long and prosper.

No Thinking & No Kidding

Boot camps or intense workout like HIIT classes (high-intensity interval training) might be a better fit. If you like being yelled at and spurred on to squeeze out every bead of sweat and burn those extra calories, this is for you. You don't have to think because there will be a coach there to do it for you. All you have to do is work it out. These are also usually done in a group setting with a coach leading the charge.

No Time!

There are certain moves you can do at your desk. Instead of a coffee break or a snack, do some push-ups off the side of your desk, or dips in your chair to work out biceps and triceps. A quick walk up and down the stairs for five minutes. Take a long way around to a college's desk.

Make sure you are getting up every hour and doing something. It is not good for your circulation to sit hour after hour.

Yo No Tener Dinero!

No money, no problem. You can always do squats and lunges across the yard. Get some free weights and work on your arms. Walk or jog in your neighborhood. Start a walking group after work with friends and co-workers. There are many options. You can also sign-up for a local run and use that as a goal for training.

There are so many options to choose from: dog walking, playing with your kids, city classes, gyms, jazzercise, yoga, swimming, water aerobics, belly dancing, off the couch Wii Fit games, ballroom dancing, the list goes on.

So get out there and get moving. You can do this.

Mood Booster!

Depression can be marked by a range of feelings from loneliness to absolute despair. You may find yourself screaming or crying for no reason. We will look at the connection between stress, anxiety, and the release of hormones and how that affects the body in a minute. But first, let's look at how exercise can actually lift us out of these blue moods and give us another tool to get going when we are stuck.

Endorphins are an example of a positive trigger. Your body releases endorphins and reduces stress hormones such as cortisol when you exercise. Endorphins are built-in "happy pills" people talk about. With exercise, you get a cocktail of high spirits in the form of dopamine, serotonin, and adrenaline. These happiness hormones can pull most of us out of mild depression. If you find yourself sliding sideways into a bad place. Try to stop it in its tracks by taking a quick fifteen-minute power walk.

Pets and Peace

If you don't have a furry friend, you might want to think about adopting a cat or a dog. Studies show that after a stressful task, the lowest stress response tested with the quickest recovery time were those of owners with their pet and only their pet. Even if they had a spouse and the spouse and the pet were both with the test subject, they didn't recover as fast. The one-on-one pet-owner bond was the strongest for stress relief.

Another study reported that spending a short amount of time with a therapy dog helped patients with upcoming operations reduce stress levels by almost 40% more than patience with no interaction. Pets are a powerful source of stress relief. The bond can help reduce blood pressure, lower levels of cortisol and elevate your happiness hormones. And you always have a willing exercise bud with Fido at your side!

Forgive and Support Yourself

Everyone falls off the wagon, it's going to happen. Don't let it spin into a worry loop, forgive yourself and hop back on. Forgiving yourself and moving on isn't as easy as it sounds and requires kindness, compassion, and understanding.

Give voice to the mistake and acknowledge it out loud. Think about what emotions you were feeling when you stumbled. How do you feel now? Like we discussed earlier, a mistake is simply a learning experience. Don't dwell on the fact that you faltered but learn from the episode. Do not allow the mean-mouth to crank up. Being self-deprecating is not going to serve you well. Review all you have done and be proud of what you have accomplished.

Remember the construction scenario. Your past does not define you and each day you have a chance to start new. There was one case where a person with PTSD felt irreparably damaged. This had built up over years and this person had no idea they had a diagnosis of PTSD until a complete breakdown lead them to the right counselor. Learning to be in the present and see themselves as the person they were at the time of the trauma was a huge mountain to climb and get over, but they did.

But it didn't happen overnight. It took time to change the mental image this person had of themselves. The counselor told them to think of themselves as something beautiful that needed protecting, caring, and nurturing. Whenever negative thoughts or images appeared, they were to shield their inner self and not let the negative through.

This person became his own bodyguard and nurtured the small child or flower or whatever he pictured, deep inside. This image helped the adult feel strong an ability to protect himself even though he was left unprotected all those years ago.

After some time the image of the beautiful inner self became on with this person's mental image of himself. Very empowering and healing. You can forgive and support yourself.

~ Oh, how I've envied the lives of those who could spend life sitting down. A place to sit, a place to sit! I'd lament, circling my empty chair. ~

- Wolfgang Hilbig, The Tidings of the Trees.

Physical Effects of Overthinking

Let's connect the dots between emotional responses, anxiety, and stress. Anxiety is a natural reaction to stressful situations. Stress comes about as a natural part of the demands and pressures we feel each day. Traffic delays, interruptions at work, emergencies that wreck our carefully crafted schedules, or chronic aches and pains are examples of situations that can cause stress in our everyday lives.

Stress can be broken down into two parts. The first part is the perception of a challenge which, in turn, triggers the second part known as "fight or flight". These responses are a result of our lineage at a time when our ancestors were on the menu of local predators. Today's challenge comes in the form of an irate driver, crabby co-worker, a child with the flu, or pulled muscles from too much workout and not enough warm-up.

There are a number of physical problems triggered when overthinking reaches the point of constant worry and anxiety. The "fight or flight" response leads to the release of stress hormones such as cortisol. The result can be elevated blood sugar and triglyceride (fat in the blood) levels. Other possible physical reactions are:

Tremors

Sweating

Dry mouth

Lack of concentration

Muscle aches and tension

Fatigue

Irritability

Digestive disorders

The onset of coronary artery disease

Possible heart attack

As stated earlier, left untreated chronic worrying can lead to depression and even thoughts of suicide. Stress is an example of a physical trigger rather than an emotional trigger. It is important to understand this because a great deal of your success depends on you being about to avoid emotional and physical triggers as you face various challenges throughout the day.

There is a difference between the hard-work ethic most American's were raised with and a constant grind that leaves you drained emotionally and physically. Our relatives worked hard to build America, but they knew how to play hard and relax, as well. Somewhere along the way, we have lost the ability to make play and relaxation a part of our normal day. We work it into our schedule as "vacation time" or downtime is reserved for Father's Day, Mother's Day, or Christmas vacation.

Think about your day and figure out where you can schedule in some relaxation in the form of 15 minutes of deep breathing, listening to calming music, or taking a quick, brisk walk. Do that twice a day and it will make a difference. Perhaps you can introduce a 2:30 p.m. espresso shot club at work. A fifteen-minute break where everyone brings their demitasse cups and socializes while caffeinating to beat the afternoon slump.

Fear of Failure

Shutting off the overthinking, worrying, and anxiety is all about building confidence. We have addressed the meaning of overthinking and anxiety. Completed exercises to help uncover the root cause of the anxiety. Looked at what might trigger worry loops and other stressors. Discussed physical and emotional health and needs. All to build confidence that you can identify coping mechanisms to stop most of these worries before they become chronic anxiety.

Now let's focus on keeping your confidence high when things don't go as planned. Don't let the fear of failure become another situation that shuts you down and prevents you from succeeding with your endeavors.

When you try and fail, you learn something about yourself and what you are trying to achieve. A failed job interview could mean you need more experience or training. It might mean you need to spend more time researching the company or practice interviewing with a friend. It doesn't mean that you are a failure.

Failure can make us feel both fear and shame. What will our friends and family think of us? They're right; I'll never amount to anything - the mean-mouth strikes again. **You don't feel smart enough and can't see yourself in that position so why did you try?**

Take a good look at what you did to prepare for the task at which you failed. Was there some self-sabotage? Did you do all you could to prepare and/or train for the job/task? Touch base with a trusted friend and discuss what you could have done differently. Figure out where the breakdown was in your preparation and fix it. You need to own the fear by turning failure into a positive learning experience. You will do better next time.

Another confidence builder understands what is under your control. Was it a lack of preparation or not having the right connections? You can change the dynamics and control both of those situations. Research, education, and training will help with preparation. Building your contact network by mining your social media network for friends who might be able to help you connect with the right people.

~ Is there a place you can go to break away for a little while? If you haven't yet built your treehouse, it's never too late to start. ~

- Gina Greenlee, Postcards and Pearls: Life Lessons from Solo Moments on the Road

Take a Breather

Please take time out to reflect on what you have accomplished to this point and appreciate the work you have done so far - which is quite a bit.

You have learned exactly what overthinking is and how it differs from other anxiety disorders. You have learned the signs of an over-thinker and how to document the various loops that take up time and real estate in your head. That's a huge step in itself to realize how expensive those worry loops are when you look at what else you could be doing with that time.

You have learned to recognize triggers and found meaning in the connections of the trigger to the worry loops. You have learned coping strategies for getting your good night's sleep back. For shutting off the mean-mouth loop full of negative chatter.

You have learned how to recognize stress-inducing relationships and how to avoid them or set boundaries to keep them at a safe distance. You have learned to cherish and nurture the friends and family who already support you, and not burden them with problems out of their skill sets.

You have learned coping mechanisms for clutter management, keeping your workplace comfortable and welcoming (to you). You are taking better care of your physical health with a better diet, exercise, and a hard look at any self-medicating or self-sabotage.

You acknowledge the physical effects of overthinking and are alert for any signs that may be affecting your health and welfare. You have learned to look at failure as a lesson and speak to your fear so that it does not under-mind you.

So take a little time off to let the information soak in so that new, healthy habits lock in place. Only a day or two. It won't kill the momentum, because you have your daily routines in place for journaling as you become aware of triggers or negative thoughts. After your short break, we will start with chapter six and pull together our action plan.

Chapter 8: Remove Negative Thoughts

And Negative Influence

We, human beings, view the entire world via our mental makeup and attitude. If, in any case, this attitude of our mind turns out to be negative predominantly, it can actually impact everything in your life, which also includes your health, family, career, and various other aspects of your life. Along with that, negative thoughts come with a spiraling kind of effect, which attracts more amount of negative thinking. Negativity which wells up inside us or in our surroundings can quickly turn out to be very toxic in nature, and it can also hold us back from living the kind of life which we actually want. Luckily, you can slowly train your inner-self with time on how you are supposed to think by the implementation of very easy and simple techniques.

Techniques for getting rid of negative thoughts

Let's have a look at some of the techniques.

Having regular time for negative thoughts: It can be regarded as a paradoxical kind of strategy for gaining control over your negative form of thinking by committing around ten minutes every day for reviewing and ruminating all your negative thoughts over and over again. NTT or negative thought time needs to be for at least 10 minutes and also needs to be practiced every day. When you are having any sort of negative thought during the course of your day, try to jot it down and ask yourself that you will be reviewing the same during your NTT. With time, you will be able to gain complete control over your negative thinking, and it will also be stopping eventually.

Replacing all your negative thoughts: You cannot overcome your negative form of thinking, but you can actually replace them. For most of the individuals, the patterns of negative thoughts are well-worn pathways of neural nature. It comes with four very simple and easy steps:

Properly notice the time as you start the pattern.

Acknowledge that it is the very pattern that you want to be changed.

Articulate all the aspects which you want to be in a different form.

Choose a different kind of behavior, the behavior which you feel actually serves your target or goal.

Being your own best friend: Human beings are the meanest to themselves. Almost 90% of the self-talk is of a negative nature. You are required to follow three steps for overcoming this:

Release all that you have. Let the negative thoughts out for helping the process and not for dwelling with it.

Track it down. Properly identify when you are actually having negative thoughts.

When you become aware of your negative patterns, it will be helping in reframing all your thoughts.

Reframe all of your negative thoughts. Once you have understood it clearly why you are so mean to yourself, try to think what your best friend will be telling you in such a moment. Then just tell your inner-self all those things which you actually need to listen to.

Writing in place of just thinking: Try to write down why your negative thoughts are present. When you replace thinking with writing, it helps in purging out all your thoughts out, and when you are able to see all the words on a piece of paper or on a screen, it will become easier for you to make sense out of the same and then just move forward with it.

Making conscious efforts for finding out things to like, love and appreciate: Instead of just fighting all your negative thoughts, you can reach out consciously for the thoughts which can make you feel a lot better. One of the powerful ways of doing this by speaking out loud, if possible, by you to what you like love and appreciate. Are you heading into a tough kind of thought? "I really love the taste of coffee today", "I really like the way of seating out here", "I would appreciate all the chances of processing all these ideas with my team". Such statements to yourself can help you in reaching out for the relief, and you can find it also very easily.

Asking yourself tough natured questions: You can reflect all your answers on some tough kind of questions.

What do I actually receive in life with these patterns of negative thinking?

What am I getting as a reward for this?

What am I losing in life for engaging myself in the negative nature of thoughts?

What will I gain from positive thinking?

What is the reason behind the patterns of negative thinking?

What am I supposed to do now?

When you question yourself all of these, you can easily find the answer to your solution.

Establishing new kind of habits: Rather than just thinking of the process in terms of overcoming all your negative thoughts, you can think of the same in terms of establishing some new kind of habits. You can achieve this by directing all your senses and attention to those subjects where there is no requirement of overcoming anything. These could include subjects which you already feel nice about, and thus you can think of the subject in a positive way. The subject could be your very own pet, your love for traveling, your liking for being on the beach, etc. You can always start with something which is very easy by nature.

Prevent yourself from watching the early morning news: It has been found from various studies that even 3 minutes in the morning of negative news can easily increase your very chances of a negative kind of experience over the natural course of your day. It has also been found that the positive nature of mindset can easily improve your productivity and can also provide you with satisfaction along with reducing your rates of making errors. Mindset is your very own choice but might not be an easy thing always. Look out for eliminating all the negative form of influences from your life and also stop watching the morning bulletin or news.

Using affirmations: As you wake up every day and open your eyes, try to feel the gratitude for a fresh new day. You can write down affirmations daily, such as: 'I love all the people whom I work with,' 'I try to make positive nature of contributions every day' or 'I am always open for inspiring thoughts.' In case any negative thought creeps in your mind, try to think of a success which you have achieved recently along with the feeling which you experienced at that moment.

Positive thinking is a daily form of the task but is also worth all the results.

Developing the success routine: You can do this by taking out some amount of time every morning as you wake up and then meditate. You are required to focus on the kind of person which you actually want to become in your life along with the great quality of life which you have been planning to live in the future. You are required to set up some new sort of goals for keeping up with the momentum of building up slowly in the direction of your dream. When you actually have the idea about what you want from life, and you are constantly trying to achieve the same, you will see that negativity will slowly fade away from your mind.

Channeling all the negative thoughts into something productive: The patterns of negative thoughts can take over easily, but a great trick is to properly identify the pattern of your negative thinking along with a job that you are really excited about. Every time when you find out that you are focusing only on the negatives, try to refocus all your thoughts for a period of 10 minutes on your very new project which you are excited about. You can easily channel all your negative kind of thoughts into your new project.

Focusing only on gratitude: Gratitude is often regarded by most of the people as being underrated, but in actual, it is very important for leading a happy life. Life isn't going to become easier, but you will become stronger day by day as you learn to reframe all your difficulties in your life by identifying all the little sort of things which is actually going around you. You can keep up with a good list and try to refer to the same daily. Try to focus on the things which you really want in your life and also try to be very specific when you identify your goals. A focused and positive kind of mind will easily attract what it actually wants over time.

Try out meditation: It is not possible for anyone to escape from their negative thoughts unless and until you disrupt them physically. For getting all your negative thoughts out of your mind, you are required to get into your own body. You can do this by opting for breath work for a period of 10-15 minutes, or body movements such as yoga can help in disrupting all your negative thoughts. Yoga and meditation come with proven powers of positivity, and it can readily help in calming all your senses so that you can concentrate on positive kind of thinking.

Not paying attention to what others will say: When you start concentrating on what other people will say about you if you do something or do not do something can readily impart negative thoughts in your mind. In such situations, you are most likely to zap all your personal form of power and fall in the trap of analysis paralysis. When you actually get stuck in all such thoughts, you will actually drag yourself much more away from reality. The truth is that people around you do not have that much time, energy or attention for thinking or talking about anything that you do. People around you have their own world where they have their pets, kids, jobs, families along with their very own worries and fears.

This sort of realization or rather a reminder can really help you in setting yourself free from all the constraints which you are most likely to build up in your mind and will also help you in taking the required steps for achieving what you actually want in your life. In case people say anything about you, try not to pay attention and enjoy your own way of living your life.

Questioning your thoughts: The best thing that can be done on your part when negative thoughts tap on your shoulder and tries to grow in your mind is to just question the thought. Just ask yourself: 'Should I take these thoughts in a serious way?'. This will often lead you to answers where you are not required to pay any sort of attention to the negative sort of thoughts. When you are tired or hungry or get overworked, negativity can easily crop up in your mind. Try to focus all your inner answers on the positive aspects of your life. You might also come across answers from your inner-self when you find that just because you have made a small mistake, that does not mean that you will be getting the whole thing wrong. When you question your thoughts, you are actually performing a reality check.

Replacing negativity in the surroundings: All the things which you allow into your mind each and every day will actually have a big effect on your life. Try to figure out the sources of negativity in your life. It might turn out to be any person, magazine, website, music, and various other things. Try to ask yourself what can be done by you for spending the least amount of time with the sources of negativity in your daily life. When you can successfully analyze the sources of negativity in your life, you will be able to distance them away from you. You will be able to see the results readily where you are most likely to find yourself as a completely changed person.

Stop creating mountains from the molehills: For the very purpose of stopping a very small negative kind of thought from taking the shape of a huge monster in your very mind, try to comfort the same at the earliest as possible. Try to analyze the thoughts with questions like is it going to matter to you in the next 2 years of your life? When you find out that you have been actually creating a mountain from a molehill, you can easily get away from the negative thoughts which have been building up in your mind.

Talk it over: When you start piling up all the negative thoughts in your mind without letting anyone know about the same, you are actually doing great harm to yourself. Try to let all your negative thoughts out by talking about the same with someone close to you. When you just vent the thoughts only for a few minutes, it can actually help in seeing the overall situation in new lights. If you cannot have a conversation about your negative thoughts with someone, try to have some positive kind of conversation, which can help in boosting up the positive side of your mind.

Not letting in the vague fears: One of the most common types of mistake which most of the people make when it comes to the aspect of fear is that they become very scared of the same and try to run away from the very situation instead of just giving it a closer look and trying to fight it over. It is actually very natural when you feel this sort of impulse, but when the fears are actually vague in nature, they might turn out to be scarier than they really are. Try to examine the situation like: What is the worst that could happen in this situation? When you actually realize the result of the fear and figure out that the end result isn't that bad as you think, you can easily fight it over. You can also start to opt for listing and taking various actions of a few of the things in your life which could actually decrease the very likelihood of the worst scenarios from taking place. You can easily gain clarity about the very situation and can gain all the strength that you need for fighting over the fear.

Negativity and patterns of negative thoughts are destructive in nature. It can actually ruin your way of living or the goals which you want to achieve. If you find yourself in situations where negative thoughts are filling up your mind, take action immediately, and try to use the mentioned techniques for fighting it over.

Chapter 9: Declutter Your Mind

Clutter in the mind is one of the main reasons why people worry. When you already have a lot of things in your mind, there is absolutely no way you could get rid of worry. When your mind is cluttered, it means that it is congested. Clutter in the mind does not only increase worry, but it also gets in the way of clear thinking and focus. Before thinking of how to get rid of worry completely, it is essential that you clear your mind of all sorts of clutter. When you successfully do that, it will be easier to know what is bothering you so that you can successfully tackle worry.

How exactly do you declutter your mind? There are a lot of methods that help people declutter their minds. Some of these methods may not work for everyone, so it is essential that you pick the one that best suits you. Some of these methods include:

1. Learning to write things down:

Writing things down is probably one of the best ways to declutter your mind. Your mind may be full of things like schedules, phone numbers, appointments, and so on. You could use an app on your phone or an online tool to help you get certain things down. It should be something that will remind you from time to time about what you need to get done and when you need to get it done. When you have a way to store random significant information, it will take that stress away from your brain, thereby reducing clutter. You may think that this would not be effective, but it is. For instance, when you put the ideas of your future projects in a place where you can find it without actually stressing yourself to remember, you stand a chance of worrying less. When you always look for something important over and over again, you get stressed, and when you get stressed, you start getting worried, all because you did not have a way to declutter your mind correctly.

You could try this method with apps that send reminders to you once in a while but not every time—just enough to make sure that you know what you have set aside to do.

2. Declutter your physical space:

It is said that physical clutter often leads to mental clutter. Your brain is being reminded by your physical clutter that there is something else that needs to be done even when there is nothing. When you have this constant issue around you, how can you get rid of worry? Physical clutter hits the mind every time with a lot of stimuli, which makes the brain work overtime. When your brain works overtime, easy activities will prove difficult and challenging activities will prove impossible.

If you want to declutter your mind, you should first of all check if there is any clutter around you, maybe in your bedroom, your kitchen, or even your office. If you do not get rid of the clutter around you, there is no way you are going to get rid of the clutter in your mind.

Many people try to declutter their minds by trying a lot of things. After some time, they give up because none of the methods they have adopted actually work. It is imperative to know that those methods would have worked if they had seen what was right in front of them. There is no way any decluttering techniques can work for you when you have more physical clutter than mental clutter.

3. Make a journal:

There is a slight similarity between making a journal and writing things down, but journals are where you write your more precise thoughts. When you have a journal, you could write about things that interrupt your thinking every time. There is no actual required time for writing in your journal. You can write in it anytime you feel uneasy or you feel like your mind is full or even anytime you want to declutter your mind. You can write about things that you are worried about.

Most times, people worry without actually knowing what they are worried about, maybe because the worries are too much for them or because they can't remember. When you have a journal, you can write about your worries as soon as they hit you. This way, you will be able to tackle them one by one without actually stressing yourself about what you need and what you don't. You could also write some plans for achieving a particular goal. When you have a goal in mind, it is crucial that you write your plans for achieving that goal in your journal. This way, your mind has the time to handle other issues that come to it without going back to check on your plans. You could carry your journal from time to time to remind yourself about what you need to do to get to your goals.

Finally, you could write about any energy-zapping relationships. Relationship issues are one of the main things that clutter minds, especially when that issue looks unsolvable. You could write this in your journal as well. Try to weigh out the pros and cons of everything and see if it is worth your time and energy. If it's not, it is vital that you send that relationship out the window because it is creating unnecessary clutter. It is filling up space where there could be innovative and creative ideas and thoughts.

4. Avoid multitasking:

Multitasking is excellent and all, but not when you are trying to get rid of clutter in your mind. When you multitask with a lot of clutter in your mind, you are bound to break down. How can you do more than two things at once when you barely have space for one in your mind? When you have a lot of things to do, make sure that you make time for each and every one of them. Some people might think that they can still multitask even with a lot on their minds, but you must know that even if you do, there is no way you are going to get everything done correctly.

For instance, you could decide to tidy the kitchen and make breakfast for your kids at the same time. If your mind is cluttered, there is a considerable chance that your kids may be eating pancakes with no sugar, and there is also a possibility that your phone might end up inside one of the kitchen cabinets as well. You are not superhuman. You need to organize, and that can only be done when you have a clear mind that is free of clutter and worry.

5. Forget about the past:

You need to let go of anything from your past that hinders your future endeavors. This may be mistakes, hurt feelings, lost opportunities, and lots more. The bottom line is that these things should not create unnecessary clutter in your mind. There are a lot of people that have big boxes of bad memories in their minds—memories that take up space where good ideas should be. When these memories hold you back, there is no way you will be able to get rid of mental clutter, which means that you will be letting both the things in the past and the things in the present make you worry.

All you have to do at this point is to pick a day for yourself. A day when you will do nothing and will not be disturbed. When you have that day, take your time to go through those bad memories and discard as much as you possibly can. This may seem difficult or impossible, but it is not. You can choose to forget certain things if you want them forgotten. You have to focus on what matters and when you do, you will notice that your mind will be a lot less crowded, and you will be able to focus more on the things in front of you and less on the things of the past.

The past can be significant. It shows us the bad things we did before so that it does not repeat itself, but when it is taking up more space than it should, it is essential that you throw it out of your mind and make room for the things that you need. When you have experienced something painful, you do not need a constant reminder.

6. Restrict the amount of information that comes into your brain:

A lot of information can easily take up unnecessary space in your brain. When you need to declutter your mind, you must limit the amount of information that comes into your mind. This includes information from TV shows, magazines, blogs, or any social media activity. Your mind is already at its limit in terms of space; you do not need to clog it even further with unnecessary things. You need to stop taking in information that you know that you don't need or would never need. Instead of taking junk information, you could take in information that will help you a lot in finding what you want, which is a decluttered mind.

You can easily create space in your brain by doing the following:

Limit the time you spend on social media: Not a lot of people are going to be happy with this. Some people are social media addicts without actually knowing it. When you spend all your time on social media, you tend to soak up a lot of relevant and irrelevant information at the same time, and things that you know add no benefit to your life. If you are on different social media platforms like Instagram, Facebook, Twitter, and so on, it is imperative to stick to just one for now. When you do pick that one, try as much as you can to spend a limited amount of time on it. If you are used to spending hours on them, try spending minutes instead.

Decide what is relevant: You do not have to deceive yourself by saying that something irrelevant is relevant. You are a human being that can reason. All you have to do is look at everything you are doing and quietly decipher the things that are relevant and the things that are not. When you have successfully sorted out the relevant from the irrelevant, you must discard the irrelevant because they are the ones clogging up your brain. Take your phone for example. After a period of usage, you notice that the space in it has reduced, and you tell yourself that you have nothing literally in the phone to take up space but when you sit down and check, you notice that you have unnecessary things in there and when you remove those things, your phone memory becomes free. The same principle applies to the decluttering of your mind.

Cancel subscriptions from blogs and magazines: You should cancel subscriptions from magazines and blogs that add no value to your life. Why would you want to keep subscriptions for magazines on how to grow chest hair when that is the least of your problems? If you must keep those subscriptions, it should be magazines or blogs that motivate you and take you to places that help you. This is what you should be looking for when trying to subscribe to a new magazine or blog.

Pay attention to relevant people: You should not pay attention to just anyone that you see or anyone that everyone is paying attention to because if you do, you will be storing unnecessary information without you knowing it. If you must listen to anything someone has to say, make sure that thing is completely relevant. It could be a piece of advice, opinion, and so on. When you create space in your brain and only take in the relevant information from relevant individuals, there is no way you will have unnecessary clogs.

7. Make some of your routine decisions without thinking:

Small everyday decisions can take a lot of space in the brain, but this can easily be avoided by putting certain decisions on autopilot. Decisions that you know that do not need a lot of thought. Decisions like what you and the family will have for breakfast the next day. It is essential to plan, but if this is the least of your problems, allow it to work itself out the next day. If you cannot stay calm without making plans about breakfast, you should make your plans as short and precise as possible. Do not go into a lot of detail because when you do, you fill your brain with things that should not be there.

Another thing you should put on autopilot is deciding what to wear each day. This is something that almost everyone does, especially if they have an important event to go to. There have been reports of people that start picking out dresses for an occasion a week before, and it's still not enough time for them. Those people probably have little or nothing to worry about, but you don't. When you spend a lot of time thinking about what you will wear, or what color combination would best suit you, you will be stressing yourself unnecessarily. The time, energy, and effort you use in doing that could have been used for something more productive and effective. When you wake up in the morning, you should go to your wardrobe and pick out something that will soothe you. It doesn't need a lot of thought. When you make these kinds of decisions without thinking, it frees up a lot of space, making assimilation easier and more effective.

Finally, making decisions on what you will have later in the day, maybe for lunch, is another thing that fits perfectly in this category. These are things that should not bother you a lot. When you want to do something like make lunch, all you have to do is to make an essential list of all you need, then go to the store to get them. You don't need to start overthinking things. If you succeed in making some of these small decisions without having to go around your house walking back and forth like a mad person, you will notice that your mind will feel relaxed and more open, which means that it will be free of clutter and when your mind is free of clutter, there's absolutely no way you will worry a lot.

8. Always be decisive:

There are a lot of people in the world that find it hard to make individual decisions. Some of them do not even worry about anything but still find it hard to make certain decisions. These decisions may be important or irrelevant as the case may be, but the bottom line is that they can't just decide.

For instance, if your mailbox was filled with letters and papers, and you can't decide on what to do with them, what do you think would happen? Your mailbox would overflow with bills, letters, and so on. This could have been avoided if you just made certain decisions that would have removed them. If you want to clear that box, you must make decisions about what to do with every paper in that box. The same principle applies to the mind.

The mind is like a box that takes in a lot of information daily. If you do not know what to do with all of that information, it is only going to keep entering the brain until there is no more space for it anymore. You must make decisions about the information that you get every day. When you get home after a long day, process everything that was absorbed by your brain, then discard the irrelevant information. When you learn to sort important mail from irrelevant mail, you will notice that your brain will feel less clogged and it will be easier for you to make certain decisions.

9. Meditation is key:

You need to learn meditation because it is one of the most effective ways of getting rid of mental clutter. Meditation is not very easy for a lot of people because of their schedule or the environment they live in. Meditation needs a tranquil and calm environment. When you have that, you are halfway there. Then you have to create time for your meditation because it is not something that should be rushed. If you rush meditation, there is no way you will get anything out of it. When you have created time for meditation, all you have to do is focus your mind on only present moments. This may take a lot of time, depending on how much clutter you have up there. This is why it is important to create as much time for meditation as possible. When you can successfully focus on the things of the now, the things that are relevant and forget about the things that are not, you will be able to declutter your mind just by sitting down and focusing on something as small as your breathing.

It is said that when you meditate to clear clutter, it is like taking your mind through a car wash and at the other side, only the important things remain while the things that aren't get washed away. If you want to get the most out of all of this, you must clear your mind of certain things first. Also, this meditation will not work if you are skeptical about it. You must believe that something will work before wanting it to work for you. If you do not think that meditation will work, there is no need for you wasting your time and trying it.

10. Learn to prioritize:

Most people tend to have an endless to-do list in their minds at all times. This is one of the reasons why clutter forms in the first place. You should look at yourself and accept that there is no way you are going to get everything done at once. When you get to agree with yourself, then all you have to do is to focus on the things that you consider extremely important. Make shorter and more achievable lists, and when you do that, it will free up space in your mind, which means that your mind is decluttered.

11. Learn to breathe:

A lot of people would be like, "But I breathe." Yes, you do, but you do not breathe properly. When was the last time you actually stopped whatever you were doing or thinking about and just took a very deep breath? If you check, it has probably never happened. Taking a deep breath once in a while is an excellent way to clear your mind and free your brain from any clutter that might be taking up space. Breathing correctly helps to elevate your mood and induce tranquility.

There are a lot of people out there with constant bad moods. This may be because they have not had time to breathe and clear their minds of whatever is in there. When your mind is free of everything bad, there is no way you can be in a bad or sad mood.

Taking deep breaths also helps reduce blood pressure and heart rate, which helps the body to relax at all times. When you want to declutter your mind, you must do it when you are relaxed, and breathing is one of the sure ways of doing that. Some of us are missing out on things like this because we are always in haste, rushing to get things done. When you do that, you are only adding to what you already have in your head. Stop sometimes and breathe a little. It doesn't mean that it should take all of your time; it could be for a minute or thirty seconds depending on how long you want it to be. The bottom line is that you need to make sure that you breathe.

12. Learn to share:

Share your thoughts and whatever is bothering you with someone you trust. It may be a friend or family member. A problem shared, they say, is half solved. When you learn to share whatever is bothering you with someone, they tend to tell you what you need to do at that point. Sometimes after the talk, the problem is completely eradicated. Other times, it is not but it would feel good actually to get it off your chest.

When you have a severe problem like relationship issues, it is imperative that you share it with someone that you trust as soon as possible for you to get it out of your mind because if you don't, you might end up doing something silly or stupid and later regret it. If you want to solve your problem, you need to do it with a clear head, and if you do not have a clear head, there is no way you can solve that problem. Sometimes, it is good to get a therapist to help you clear your head because they will have a lot more experience in the matter. If you do this correctly, at the end of all this, you will have a clear and decluttered mind.

13. Take some time off to unwind:

This is the last of all the methods of decluttering. Your mind may be referred to as a machine, but it also needs to get a lot of rest. Your mind needs as much rest as possible. You need to create time for your mind to rest at all times. It doesn't mean that you have to take out two or three days to unwind. You need to make it like a vacation for you and your mind alone. You should pick a location that is very calm and quiet, a place where you will not be disturbed in any way. When you know that you have such a place, all you have to do is take your gadgets like your phones, tablets, and computers and turn them off. The main aim here is to stay away from the outside world and what they have to say. When you succeed in doing this, you will notice that your mind will be more open to specific ideas and thoughts.

If you do not want to travel or pick a location far from home because of your kids, you could decide to take a long walk in the park when the kids are in school, or you could choose to take a long, well-deserved nap. Before you do any of these two things, you must come out with a clear mind. Come outside with a mind that wants to be free of clutter. Do not just do all of this because people say it is good for you, do it because you know it is right for you.

Clearing the mind of every kind of clutter is something that not a lot of people are aware of. Some people sit in their houses every day with constant worry and uneasiness, not knowing what is causing it. Little do they know that what is causing the problem is right in front of their very eyes. When you know what is wrong with you, you will be able to tackle the problem, but when you don't, there is no way in the world, you will be able to because you can only solve a problem when you know what that problem is.

Chapter 10: The Key For Inner Peace:

Meditation

6.1 What Is Meditation?

Don't like the idea of sitting in silence and breathing for half an hour? What is the point of meditation anyway? Before you dismiss meditation as a form of treatment for anxiety- read this chapter!

Meditation is not all about reducing stress or letting go and taking a few moments for ourselves to try and recompose and regain our thoughts. Meditation is about more than that.

It is about finding balance, inner peace and calm in a world where it seems almost every aspect of our lives is capable of triggering stress, worry or anxiety. Our bodies and minds may be strong and tough, but there is only so much negativity that it can take before it starts to take its toll and affect our health, sometimes to a point where it could become unbearable.

If only there were a magic formula of some sort where we could keep out these negative feelings that are capable of causing such destruction within our minds and bodies, but there isn't. Which is why we need to turn to meditation as a way of managing our worries and anxieties, to find a way to find that balance within ourselves and recharge our energy.

The beauty of meditation is that it is simple yet powerful. Simple enough that anyone can learn how to do it effectively with the right tools, teachings, and techniques. Anyone can learn the art of meditation, and it isn't as difficult as you may imagine. Sure, you may have tried it a few times and found yourself struggling in the early stages to quiet your mind and achieve a focus, calm, and mindful state, but that is perfectly normal, especially if you're a beginner just starting out on this journey.

Mastering the art of meditation, like everything else, takes patience, time and practice. You're putting far too much pressure on yourself if you expect to get it right from the moment you sit cross-legged on your mat and shut your eyes hoping to achieve deep meditation right from the get-go. No, it takes time and practice, and you need to be patient with yourself. In this book, you will find a four-week plan that will help you achieve deep meditation, and the key to succeeding in this is to remember that you need to be patient. Practice makes perfect, which is why your goal of achieving deep meditation is spread out over four weeks, you need time to master each stage and phase of the process before moving onto the next. With repeated effort and your goal clearly in mind, you will see results at the end of the four weeks.

6.2 Why Meditation?

Is it just about calming our minds and finding inner peace? One part of it yes, that is why a lot of people find meditation to be a helpful practice. Those who avidly do this find that their mind is peaceful and free from worries and mental discomfort, making it easier for them to achieve happiness compared to those who do not practice meditation at all. If you've never tried it, you may scoff at the idea of how sitting quietly for a few minutes every day is going to make a difference in your life, but you would be surprised.

Think about it. What is it that successful people and motivational speakers often say they do as part of their daily routine? That's right, they spend a few hours meditating in the morning. Clearly, it's working for them, isn't it? Because they're able to go through life, even with the struggles that may come their way, with a positive attitude and they don't let stress get the best of them.

Now, you don't necessarily have to practice meditation in the morning the way they do, you can meditate and anytime that works best for you. There is no hard and fast rule. You can even meditate more than once a day if you need to and you find that it helps. You make your own rules according to what works best for you. By spending a few minutes each day training your mind and making meditation part of your routine, you will discover that your mind gradually is able to find peace a lot easier and finding happiness is something that doesn't seem so elusive anymore, even if you have certain challenges that you may be going through in your life. Even in the most difficult of circumstances, you will find that you're able to remain calm, steady and still be able to look at the bright side of life.

Learning to control our minds is one of the most difficult things we can do. It's easy to let our thoughts get the best of us, which is why it is so easy to be consumed by negativity and external circumstances can affect us to such an extent. The thing about this is, we don't even realize just how severely we are affected by it all because we're not really thinking too much about it. Fluctuations in our moods seem like a normal, everyday occurrence and we brush it off as being part of life and we can't control it. But that's where you would be wrong.

Because you can control it with meditation. Create that inner space and clarity in your mind that will enable you to always be in firm control of your thoughts, despite the circumstances you may be facing. Meditation is how you find that mental balance, so you're never at one extreme or the other (never too sad or never too happy). It's always about finding the right balance. You've always been told you need to live a balanced life, eat balanced meals, why not have a balanced mind too? Meditation is a way of bringing your mental clarity, and to change the way you look at the world around you.

At its very core, meditation is about taming your mind. A lot of people struggle with trying to overcome anxiety, despair, agitation and other habitual thought patterns which they may find difficult to break out of. Taming the mind through mindful meditation is how you give yourself control of your own well-being once more. Meditation will bring you a sense of fullness and completion, and believe it or not, it is the only way to truly achieve tranquillity that is easily accessible to everyone on this planet. True, there may be other temporary forms of serenity, but nothing will come close to bringing you the long-term peace that you seek no matter what you may be going through in your life the way meditation will. And what is why we learn to meditate.

Meditation has been practiced traditionally for hundreds – if not thousands- of years, it is not something that just came about overnight as a new trend. Meditation is something that is inherent in all human beings, something we all have it in us to be able to do. Many are already reaping the benefits of what meditation has to offer, and now it's time for you to start doing the same thing.

6.3 The Long Term Benefits of Meditation

The reason why most of us end up becoming stressed and anxious on a regular basis is that we do not place importance on mind and soul health. Taking care of our bodies not only means just the physical aspects of it but the mental and emotional aspects too.

Often we're just focused on taking care of the physical part of ourselves that we neglect to remember our minds need just as much attention and care because we don't realize the extent of what being weight down by stress, worry and anxiety can do it for us. These negative emotions are so powerful that in extreme cases, they can even manifest themselves physically.

Before we delve deeper into the benefits of meditation for anxiety, here are the benefits of practicing meditation consistently for your overall health and vitality:

Reduction in your stress levels

Improvement in your concentration and focus

It improves your cognitive and creative thinking skills

With greater mental clarity, you're able to make better decisions and solve problems

An increase in self-awareness

An increase in happiness

An increase in self-acceptance because meditation helps you reconnect with your inner self

It will help you learn to appreciate life more as you become more aware of your surroundings through mindfulness

You learn how to block out distractions in your life

It improves your breathing and your heart rate

Helps you feel more connected to yourself

It helps regulate your mood and anxiety disorders

Helps you sleep better at night

Helps lower your blood pressure levels

Increases serotonin production which will help improve your mood

You gain clarity and peace of mind

Your problems seem more manageable when you don't let your mind get the best of you

Increases your sense of well-being

Helps you regain emotional steadiness

It improves your mental resilience against adversity and pain

It increases your optimism

Benefits of Meditation for Anxiety

When we talk about meditation for anxiety, keep in mind that meditation is PART of the anxiety treatment. It is not meant to be a replacement for anxiety treatments prescribed by your doctor or therapist. Meditation for anxiety should be considered as a complementary treatment for anxiety and for good reason.

Research conducted in 2013 by the Wake Forest Baptist Medical Center researchers focuses on which brain regions are activated through mindfulness meditation. This research was published in the Social Cognitive and Affective Neuroscience journal. Another research also focused on generalized anxiety disorder and the benefits of meditation. This research focused on 93 individuals with DSM-IV diagnosed GAD which looked at an 8-week manualized mindfulness-based stress reduction program focusing on attention control. This program resulted in a significant reduction in anxiety for three to four study measures and participants also showed better positive self-statements.

How Meditation focuses on the mind

Consistent meditation disables the distractions we face by filtering it before it starts to bottleneck. Think of this like a river dam that ensures the right amount of water to be flowed down to households, industries, and agriculture. Meditation, in the same way, filters the less important data that we are exposed to and sends only the necessary and important info into our brain. In other words, it helps us determine what information should we focus on and what we do not need to focus on that may cause chronic anxiety.

How Meditation Reduces Cortisol

Researchers from Rutgers University and the University of California also conducted research relating to mindfulness meditation and the effects on cortisol. The study shows that consistent meditation reduced cortisol dramatically, with some results showing at least a 50% drop. Daily meditation for even 3 minutes is effective for the brain- you do not need to be a yogi with years of training to do this. Meditation is like the firefighters you call to extinguish this hormone that brings in so many diseases that can protect your health and happiness. When you do mindfulness exercises, you create an environment that is 100% inharmonious with anxiety. This mental environment prevents anxiety from manifesting in your mind and brain.

How Meditation Evolves The Brain Beyond Anxiety

A study conducted by Dr. Sara Lazar in 2005 was a landmark study that showed the brains of those who meditated were much thicker and had more folds and surface area in their prefrontal cortexes. This study is used now by various neuroscientific and psychological researches as the go-to foundational study for other mental health issues such as depression.

Those who meditation, even for 10 to 15 minutes a day are usually anxiety-free, happy and healthy. While this has been known in anxiety teachings and treatments, it is only now that modern science is recognizing the power of meditation with procuring a healthy mind and body.

Meditation Controls Anxiety through a mind-body connection

Back in the 1970s, Harvard physician Herbert Benson looked at the behaviors of the patients visiting him due to stress-related disorders such as anxiety. His observation led him to look at ways that he can counteract this association, simultaneously revolutionizing the mental care industry and helping people. Dr. Benson's discovery was the connection between the mind and body through meditation. It slowed metabolism, reduced the heart rate, resulted in measured breathing and quieter brainwave activity. All of this combined brought out the right foundations for healing.

Meditation Reverses Anxiety using relaxation

When meditating, our body activates the parasympathetic nervous system and simultaneously deactivates the body's stress mode. When this happens, the body reverses several health issues, primarily anxiety. Relating to Dr. Benson's research above, the mind-body connection gives the body the meditative state it needs to relieving anxiety and managing stress.

Why Meditation Builds Your Mindful Muscle

Yes, we have mind muscles too. Instead of constantly having knee-jerk reactions to a wide variety of craziness, silliness, and scariness that we often experience, meditation also allows you to look into the thoughts that come into your mind which you need to give your attention to, especially the thoughts and emotions that you often neglect. Our thoughts come and go and via meditation, we can at least focus on the various emotions with a more structured mind without needing to chase the rabbit down its never-ending hole. Through meditation, we can build our mental muscles and allow us to understand the deepest levels of our mind and connect to our thoughts, emotions, and mind.

How Meditation squashes Anxiety: Endorphins

Yup, that's right! It is not the only exercise that releases endorphins but also meditation. For a better mood, meditate for a few minutes after your exercise as it can bring you into a calmer, cool and happy place of your own.

When you exercise or go for a long jog, usually it gives you a natural high and joggers refer to this feeling as 'runner's high'. This zen-life state of happiness and bliss is one of the reasons why people like jogging and meditation is exactly like that except it also makes you feel calmer and it also elevates your mood.

Whenever you exercise, spend at least 5 to 10 minutes after your workouts or jog to meditate as it also helps your body come back to its normal breathing rate, allowing you to cool down both physically and mentally.

How Meditation Quiets The Mind

When you no longer overthink things or you do not have to worry or have the feeling of constant fear, or when you stop worrying endlessly about what the future holds, you get to experience a silence that is intoxicating. Meditation allows your mind to explore this side of your natural state, the stillness that is true and pure. When you meditate constantly, you eventually start to quieten your mind and stop thinking about the ticking clock, the chores you have to do and the work you need to get done. You quieten your mind to spend a few minutes in bliss and these few minutes can benefit you in a longer and more pronounced aspect of your life.

6.4 Which Type Of Meditation Is Best For You?

There are various kinds of meditations that you can try for anxiety, stress as well as panic. Just remember that meditation is just one of the things that you would be requested to do so by a health care provider or doctor. Meditation is a complementary treatment to anxiety and you should view it that way. It is not the be-all-end-all when it comes to treating anxiety because everyone's anxiety is different and it requires various different treatments for different people.

With that said, here are the different kinds of meditation that you could do to decrease your anxiety, work on your breathing as well be more mindful:

The Loving Kindness Meditation

Also known as the Metta meditation, the goal of this meditation is to cultivate an attitude of kindness and love towards everything around you, even your own enemies and also to the sources of stress. This meditation involves breathing deeply to open your minds to be more loving to their loved ones and to the people in this world. The key to this meditation is to repeat the message as often as possible until you feel an attitude of loving-kindness. This meditation is created to promote the feelings of compassion and love to oneself and the people around them. It can help in anger, resentment, and frustration as well as interpersonal conflict. You can look forward to reducing anxiety, depression as well as PTSD.

Progressive Relaxation

Also known as the body scan meditation, this meditation focuses on scanning your own body to release the areas of tension. The goal of this meditation is to notice tension in the body and also allow stress to be released. During this meditation session, you usually begin at one end of the body and work your way throughout your whole world. You can start either with your feet and work your way up or your head and work your way down.

With this meditation, you tense and relax each muscle in your body mindfully and you are also encouraged to visualize peaceful situations. Progressive relaxation can help you promote generalized feelings of relaxation and calmness and this is something that can help with chronic pain.

You will learn how to slowly and steadily relax your body and also help you sleep better.

Mindfulness meditation

This form of meditation encourages people to remain aware and present at the moment. Instead of dwelling in the past or even dreading the future ahead of you, through mindfulness meditation, it encourages awareness of your existing surroundings. Rather than reflecting on what could be or maybe, you simply live in the moment without any judgment or overthinking.

You can do this meditation anywhere, such as at your work desk, while waiting in line for coffee, at your lunch break. This enables you to calmly be aware of your surroundings, the sounds, the sights as well as the smells. Mindfulness involves being aware of your breathing as well as drawing attention to the areas of tension in your body. Research has found out that mindfulness meditation can improve focus, memory as well as reduce fixation on negative emotions and lessen impulsive emotional reactions.

The Breathing awareness meditation

This type of meditation is designed to encourage mindful breathing. It involves breathing deeply and slowly, counting breaths or focusing on breathing. The goal is to focus only on your breathing and ignore other thoughts that come into your mind. Breathing awareness also brings the many benefits of mindful meditation and it includes reducing anxiety, brings more emotional stability as well as improved concentration.

Kundalini Yoga

This type of meditation involves more yoga movements with meditation blended in with mantras and deep breathing. The best way to meditate using kundalini yoga is by learning from a teacher or joining a class. You can also learn poses and mantra through YouTube videos. Kundalini yoga not only focuses on mental strength but also physical strength, like other forms of yoga. It improves mental health by reducing depression and anxiety.

Zen Meditation

Zen meditation is a form of meditation from the practice of Buddhism. Also called Zazen, this meditation is learned from a teacher because it involves specific postures, techniques, and steps. Zen meditation requires to focus on breathing and mindful observation of your thoughts with no judgment. This type of meditation requires a quiet space to be one with only your thoughts. While it is similar to mindfulness meditation, zazen, however, needs more practice and discipline. If you want relaxation as well as spiritual guidance, zen meditation could be something you can try.

Transcendental Meditation

This is another form of meditation that has a more spiritual nature. It also involves you to be seated and to breathe in and out slowly and the goal here is to rise above or transcend your current state of being. During meditation, you need to focus on a mantra and the mantras are determined by the teachers based on the year you were born, age and other factors. People who practice transcendental meditation report having more spiritual awareness as well as heightened mindfulness.

Meditation to Relieve Anxiety

The goal for meditation to relieve anxiety is to let go of our emotions and reactions and just make an observation from a detached perspective. With meditation, you teach yourself to observe without assigning emotion to any given situation. All you need to do is observe with a blank state of mind.

Meditation also practices your mind to have a better sense of awareness of the present while still staying in control of any negativity that may come and prevent it from increasing. Meditation heightens the brain's cognitive function through mood training and mental training which can alleviate anxiety and decrease stress levels. It also teaches us to respond to reflectively and not reflexively. In doing so, not only do we prevent anxiety, but we also prevent depression and other mood disorders.

Chapter 11: Interrupt The Worry Habit

In a meeting, author and speaker Joanie Yoder shared her account of how stress almost destroyed her life—until she discovered the answer in a flash of brilliance.

"My life was full of tension and stress; however, I had the option to cover it up, as many individuals do, until I had an encounter that made me hit absolute bottom. It was then that I had to confront my tensions, my feelings of dread, my fear, and my stress.

"Catherine Marshall said that the best revelation we can make is to understand that we cannot do everything on our own; that our own qualities are insufficient. I came to that discovery on my own. I didn't have anything left of my own inward assets. I did not seem to have the ability, physically or inwardly, to go on.

"I had developed agoraphobia, which is a fear of open spaces—a dread of going out.

I most dreaded going to the grocery store. It was so serious that I would freeze and start perspiring. I was anxious about the possibility that I would go absolutely crazy in front of strangers—the feeling was beyond words.

"Here and there, I would leave the grocery store in the middle of shopping, push my truck into a corner, and run home. When I was in the house, I felt elation at being sheltered and secure once more.

"I thought that I was the only individual who felt like this. My dietary patterns changed, my rest was inconsistent, I was trembling and unstable, and I was constantly on edge about existence and every one of my duties. I couldn't confront anything. I only managed to deal with it when I was in my mid-thirties.

"There were reasons for my trouble. As I think back now, I understand that there were three explanations behind my powerlessness to oversee life:

"One was extraordinary adolescence. I was genuinely too immature to deal with my duties.

"Secondly, I had built up a propensity for sharpness. All things considered, I didn't generally realize it, although my motive was noble.

"What's more, the third reason, which I believe is normal fours all, was an inclination to act naturally adequate. I attempted to do everything on my own. What's more, even when I understood that I couldn't do it all alone, I believed I should have been able to.

"Those three components had a disintegrating impact. They drove me toward a breakdown that I required. I believe it's a breakdown that we, as a whole, need. It was everything but a mental meltdown; it was a breakdown of my independence.

"From my very own involvement, and furthermore, in watching other individuals who are in this agonizing circumstance of coming up short on their assets, one of the qualities is a need to control—the need to control life, conditions, individuals, and even God—since we feel terrified of what may occur. We feel that on the off chance that we can control things and cause things to go a specific way, we will be less apprehensive.

"My concern was that I didn't feel responsible for my self-assurance—insurance from the things that I feared. So I started to manufacture a wall around myself. That case progressed toward becoming as little as the word suggests. I had a minor space in which I had a sense of security and secure—the four dividers of my home. Truth be told, I so cased my life that it contained a populace of one—me."

Is it accurate to say that you are tormented by consistent stresses and restless contemplations?

Worries, doubts, and anxieties are a regular part of life. It's entirely expected to worry over an unpaid bill, an exceptional imminent representative gathering, or a first date. In any case, "run of the mill" worry becomes pointless when it's consistent and runs wild. You worry every day over "vulnerabilities" and unlikely scenarios; you can't dump nervous considerations out of your head, and they interfere with your daily life.

We may not all relate to Joanie's strategy for adapting; however, we, as a whole, recognize what it is to confront circumstances that make us uneasy, even panicky. A few of us stress over occupational circumstances, wellbeing, or a family that is self-destructing. Stress can appear as throbbing cerebral pain. Others experience a beating heart and brevity of breath. For still others, unrecognized dread sneaks behind our propensity to indulge, overspend, or abuse whatever will stifle the torment. We all face conditions outside our ability to control.

Frequent worrying, negative thinking, and consistently expecting the worst to happen can contrarily influence your emotional and physical health. It can, as well, zap your emotional strength, leaving you feeling anxious and apprehensive, causing insomnia, headaches, stomach issues, and muscle weight, and make it difficult to concentrate at work or school. You may take your negative emotions out on the people closest to you, self-fix with alcohol or meds, or endeavor to involve yourself by wandering off in fantasy land before screens. Excessive worrying can similarly be a huge element of Generalized Anxiety Disorder (GAD), an anxiety issue that incorporates strain, fear, and unease that goes back as far as you can recall.

If you're tormented by exaggerated worry and tension, there are steps you can take to stop anxious thoughts. Endless worry is a mental habit that can be broken. You can train your mind to stay calm and look at life from a more logical perspective while avoiding catastrophic thinking.

For what reason is it so hard to stop worrying?

Constant worrying can bring about critical harm. It can keep you up at night and make you feel tense and anxious during the day. Also, regardless of whether you despise feeling like a nervous wreck, it can be so difficult to stop. For most unending worriers, the tense thoughts are fueled by the feelings—both negative and positive—that you hold about worrying:

You may have negative feelings about anxiety. You may acknowledge that your constant worrying is ruinous, that it will make you crazy or impact your physical health. Or then again, you may be anxious that you will lose all authority over your worrying—that it will never stop. Negative feelings, or struggling with worrying, adds to your anxiety and increases worry; positive feelings about worrying can be just as harmful.

You may have positive feelings about anxiety. You may feel that your worrying is keeping you safe from fearful things, neutralizing issues, setting you up for a solution, or helping you to make plans. Maybe your belief is that if you keep obsessing about an issue long enough, you'll eventually figure it out. Or then again, perhaps you're convinced that worrying is the ideal approach to promise yourself so you won't disregard something. It's difficult to get out from under the worrying penchant unless you acknowledge that your worrying fills a positive need. At the point when you comprehend that worrying is the issue, not the solution, you can then start to regain control of your worried mind.

EXERCISE TIP 1: CREATE A DAILY "WORRY" PERIOD

It's difficult to be effective in your step-by-step practices when anxiety and worry are governing your contemplations and preventing you from concentrating on your work, school, or your home life. This is where observing your thoughts can help. Rather than endeavoring to stop or discard a tense idea, permit yourself to have it, but put off ruminating about it until later.

Make a "worry period." Choose a set time and spot to be anxious. It should be consistently available (for instance, in the family room from 5:00 to 5:20 p.m.) and early enough that it won't make you nervous right before rest time. During your anxiety period, you're allowed to worry about whatever's at the front line of your contemplations. The rest of the day is a worry-free zone.

Record your anxieties. If an anxious thought or worry comes into your head during the day, make a short note of it and, after that, continue about your day. Remind yourself that you'll have the chance to think about it later, so there's no convincing motivation to worry about it right now. Recording your insights—on a pad or your phone or PC—is much harder work than simply thinking them, so your worry will undoubtedly lose their ability.

Go over your "worry list" during the anxiety time period. If the worries that you recorded are upsetting you, make yourself worry over them, but only for the proportion of time you've allocated for your anxiety period. When you start to deal with your worries in this fashion, you'll consistently feel that it's easier to develop a more balanced perspective. Likewise, if your anxieties don't seem, by all accounts, to be critical anymore, you can cut anxiety period short and enjoy the rest of your day.

Tip 2: Challenge Restless Thoughts

If you experience the ill effects of interminable uneasiness and stress, the odds are that the way that you look at the world causes potential situations to appear more catastrophic than they really are. For instance, you may overestimate the likelihood that things will turn out unfavorably, bounce promptly to most pessimistic scenario situations, or treat each on-edge thought as though it were a certainty. You may likewise dishonor your own capacity to deal with life's issues, accepting that you'll self-destruct whenever there's any hint of an issue.

The most effective method to challenge these musings:

During your stress period, challenge your negative considerations by asking yourself:

What's the proof that the idea is valid? That it's not valid?

Is there an increasingly positive, practical method for taking a gander at the circumstance?

What's the likelihood that what I'm terrified of will actually occur? If the likelihood is low, what are some other possible outcomes?

Is this thought or idea useful? In what manner will agonizing over it help me, and in what capacity will it hurt me?

What would I say to a companion who felt this stress?

Tip 3: Distinguish Among Resolvable and Unsolvable Worries

Research shows that while you're worrying, you unexpectedly feel less nervous. Running over the issue in your brain helps you to manage your emotions because it causes you to feel that you're accomplishing something. Regardless, worrying and problem-solving are two very different things.

Problem-solving incorporates surveying a condition, creating strong steps for overseeing it, and a short time later, putting the plan in action. Worrying, on the other hand, only sporadically prompts plans. Despite how much time you spend imagining worst-case scenarios, you are not more prepared to deal with them if they should happen.

Is Your Anxiety Solvable?

Solvable worries are those you can deal with proactively right away. For example, if you're worried about your bills, you could call your loan specialist to consult him/her about your different options. Pointless, unsolvable worries are those for which there is no logically related course of action, such as worrying about the possibility of imminent disaster or envisioning a situation where your child gets into some sort of trouble.

If you are worrying about something that has a high probability of occurring, start conceptualizing. Review all the courses of action that you can take to resolve this potential problem. Take the necessary steps, but don't get too hung up on finding the perfect plan. Focus on the things that you can change, instead of the conditions or substances outside your locus of control. After you've surveyed your decision, decide on a course of action. At the point when you have a game plan and start dealing with the issue, you'll feel considerably less tense.

If the anxiety isn't actionable, recognize your helplessness. If you are a relentless worrier, most of your anxious contemplations will fall into this category. Focusing is often a possible away we endeavor to foresee what the future has in store; it is a way to deal with turn away loathsome astonishments and control the outcome. The issue is that it doesn't work. Considering all of the things in your life that could have negative outcomes won't make your life easier. Worrying about possible unlikely occurrences will simply prevent you from enjoying the many positive and helpful things that you have in the present. To stop worrying, give up your need for certainty and easy answers.

Do you, when all is said and done, catastrophically envision horrendous things will occur? What is the likelihood they will, in fact, occur?

Given that the likelihood is incredibly low, is it possible to live with the small probability that something negative may happen?

Ask your friends and family how they adjust to being able to prevent negative outcomes in similar conditions. Might you have the option to do so in like manner?

Tip 3: Talk About Your Anxieties

Talking very closely with a trusted partner or relative, someone who will listen to you without judging, denouncing, or becoming overly-involved is perhaps the best and calmest way to deal with what is occurring in your present reality and diffuse anxiety. When your anxieties start spiraling, talking them over can help you to feel validated.

Verbalizing your emotions can routinely help you to make sense of what you're feeling and put things in perspective. If your fearful emotions are also outlandish, verbalizing them can reveal them for what they are—pointless worry. Likewise, if your worries are valid, describing them to someone else can help you to create strategies to solve them that you probably would not have thought of alone.

Build a strong support system. People are social creatures; we're not expected to live in disengagement. Regardless, a strong support system doesn't generally mean a large group of friends. Having two or three people whom you can trust and rely upon to be there for you has a number of benefits. Also, if you don't feel that you have anyone to trust in, it's never too late to assemble new friendships.

Acknowledge who to avoid when you're feeling fretful. Your fretful outlook on life may be something that you developed when you were growing up. If your mother is a relentless worrier, she isn't the best individual to call when you're feeling anxious—no matter how close you are. When pondering who to go to, ask yourself whether you will, by and large, feel significantly better or even more fearful after discussing your problem or issue with that person.

Tip 4: Interrupt the Stress Cycle

On the off chance that you stress unreasonably, it can appear as though negative thoughts are racing through your mind in a permanent loop. You may feel like you're spiraling wildly, going insane, or ready to break down from carrying the weight of this unease. Be that as it may, there are steps that you can take right now to eliminate those restless musings and give yourself a break from persistent stress.

Get up and get going. Exercise is a powerful enemy of worrying and unease since it discharges endorphins, which diminish strain and stress, help vitality, and improve your feeling of prosperity. Much more critically, by truly concentrating on how your body feels as you move, you can interfere with the steady progression of stressful thoughts going through your mind. Focus on the impression of your feet hitting the ground as you walk, run, or move, for instance, or the musicality of your breathing, or the feeling of the sun or wind on your skin.

Take a yoga or jujitsu class. By concentrating your psyche on your developments and breathing, rehearsing yoga or judo keeps your focus on the present moment, clearing your brain and leading to a casual state.

Reflect. Reflection works by changing your concentration from stressing over the future or choosing not to act on to what's happening at the present moment. By being completely occupied with the present moment, you can stop the endless loop of negative considerations and stress. Furthermore, you don't have to sit leg over leg, light candles or incense, or serenade. Basically, locate a calm, agreeable spot and pick one of the many free or modest cell phone apps that can guide you through the meditation.

Practice dynamic muscle unwinding. This can enable you to break the interminable circle of stressing by concentrating your psyche on your body rather than your considerations. By first tensing, and, on the other hand, releasing diverse muscle groups in your body, you release muscle pressure in your body. Furthermore, as your body unwinds, your mind will relax as well.

Attempt profound relaxation. At the point when you start to feel stressed, you become on edge and inhale more quickly, frequently prompting further uneasiness. Yet, by breathing deeply, you can quiet your brain and calm negative contemplations.

Tip 5: Observe Your Stressful Thoughts

Stress is generally caused when we focus excessively on the future—on what may occur and what we'll do about it—or on the past, rehashing the things that we've said or done over and over in our minds. You can break free from stressful patterns of thinking by returning your focus to the present. This technique involves watching your stressful thoughts, and, after that, releasing them. Observing your stressful thoughts helps you to recognize where your reasoning is causing issues and to reconnect with your feelings.

Recognize and observe your stressful thoughts. Try not to overlook, battle, or control them like you generally would. Rather, just watch them as though from an outsider's point of view, without responding or judging.

Release your stress. Notice that when you don't attempt to control the restless musings that spring up, they pass before long, similar to mists moving across the sky. It's only when you hold in your stressful thoughts that you will start to feel paralyzed by them

Remain focused on the present. Focus on how your body feels, the pace of your breathing, your constantly-evolving feelings, and the contemplations that float through your psyche. On the off chance that you end up ruminating about a specific idea, take your consideration back to the present moment.

Utilizing mindfulness to remain focused on the present is a basic idea; however, it requires some time investment and practice to receive the rewards. From the start, you'll most likely find that your mind will meander back to your stressful thoughts. Do whatever it takes not to become disappointed. Each time that you return your concentration back to the present, you're fortifying another psychological propensity that will enable you to break free of the negative stress cycle.

Do you believe that the Universe is working with you? When you can understand this, and realize that, regardless of what you experience, eventually, everything will be fine, you will never doubt that there is a being, more powerful than you, who is ensuring that everything will be fine.

Imagine how you need your life to be and, after that, allow the Universe to work with you, knowing and expecting that it will. This will greatly reduce your stress. By attempting to change your way of thinking, you achieve a more calm, relaxed, stress-free existence.

Chapter 12: Other Factors That Supports

The Cbt Method

Learning About Anxiety

One of the first and most effective methods that are used in solving psychological problems is learning about the problem itself. This is otherwise known as psycho-education. When you learn about your problems, this will provide comfort in knowing that you are not alone in it and that there are others who were able to find strategies that helped them get over their problems.

By learning about your problems, you can also help your friends and family members because they too can gain more knowledge about your problem. Some people will discover that merely having a good understanding of their problem will be a huge boost in their journey to recovery.

Recovery Strategies

By being able to relax your body, you will also be able to boost the success of therapy. According to experts, the tension in your muscles as well as shallow breathing can be linked to both stress and anxiety and may also be one of the causes of depression, so it is a good thing to be aware of your bodily sensations. This will help you practice exercises that will help you to learn how to relax.

In CBT, calm breathing and progressive muscle relaxation are two strategies that are used for relaxation. They involve consciously slowing down one's breath and the systematic tensing and relaxation of different groups of muscles. As with all the other skills that can be practiced, the more you engage in relaxation strategies, the more effective they will be and they become more likely to work quickly. Listening to music, yoga, meditation, and massage are other relaxation strategies that could also work.

Having Realistic Thoughts

To be able to manage emotions, one has to be able to master the act of identifying negative thinking and replacing it with balanced and realistic ones. This is because our thoughts largely impact the way we feel, so if we can change our unhelpful thoughts to realistic ones, we will be able to feel much better. Having realistic thoughts, however, means having a fair and balanced view of one's self and the world without applying any form of negativity or overt positivity.

Facing One's Fears Through Exposure

It is not abnormal to want to avoid those things that we fear. This is because our fears increase anxiety for a short time. For instance, if you are one of those that harbor the fear of small-enclosed spaces like elevators, you may want to use the stairs instead because you feel like it would reduce your level of anxiety. Avoiding the things you fear, however, will not help you learn that things that you fear are not as bad as you actually think they are. In cases like this, you will not be able to learn that taking the stairs will not give you the chance to learn that taking the elevator will not result in a negative outcome.

The process used in facing one's fears during CBT is known as exposure, and this is the most important step in getting to learn effective ways of managing anxiety. This typically involves entering into feared situations repeatedly until you begin to feel less anxious about them. In the beginning, you engage in those things that make you feel a little bit of anxiety and as you proceed; you are made to face things that cause you greater anxiety.

Chapter 13: Expecting The Tide To Turn

Adrenalin Rush

People who seek scary, thrilling sports and activities are often referred to as "adrenaline junkies." For many, it becomes a true addiction. Once "hooked," these thrill-seekers will travel thousands of miles to catch the biggest waves, ski from the highest mountains, jump from airplanes, bridges, and buildings... they seek activities that trigger the release of adrenaline into their bloodstreams. After watching a program on TV that focused on such people's stories, I often wondered: what pushes them to seek these experiences again and again? I could not relate...

Living in Paradise Cove, an amazing place in Malibu known for its surf, did not motivate me to try this sport. I love to swim but the cold water of the Pacific Ocean kept me on the shore most of the time, even during the summer. As I walked on the beach, I watched surfers riding the waves in all kinds of weather condition: from gorgeous sunny days with gentle waves to stormy days and twelve-foot waves. Only a few ventured into surf when the waves resembled multi-story buildings, but those who practiced for years mastered riding the waves and fully enjoy the thrill of subduing the elements.

Anxiety can wash over as a huge, powerful and frightening wave. It is impossible to avoid waves in the ocean, and when they get extremely big it gets pretty scary. Surfers learn the patterns of the ocean currents, and for accomplished surfers, riding even the biggest swells becomes a thrilling ride. I thought that maybe I could utilize the adrenaline rush I experience during an anxiety attack and turn it into something if not pleasurable than at least not as scary.

As I was not a surfer, I thought to find another activity I can do or even imagine that will give me positive reaction to adrenaline release. I thought of watching thrillers, riding a rollercoaster or driving fast on a track, but found it in skiing. I am not an avid skier, but I can remember the thrill of going down the slopes, surrounded by the beauty of snow-covered trees, breathing the crisp mountain air. Even if I am not there, I can still imagine it. I tried it a few times when anxiety washed over: closed my eyes and imagined riding down the mountain. To my great relief, it worked. So I got another anxiety fighting, or rather in this case anxiety-utilizing tool.

As I learned what anxiety is about, what may trigger it and how I can deal with it, this adversary became less and less scary, but rather annoying.

Self-education

I had a deep desire to get well and was willing to do anything to be set free of anxiety. Switching my brain into constructive mode in the midst of immense pain was hard, but I discovered that recovery begins with the strong desire and will to get the victory. I was determined to get well and it drove me to action. I had to become proactive on my way to healing—I did not see any other way. I couldn't just sit and wait for a magic cure.

I would go to bookstores and a local library to get as many books on anxiety disorders as possible. Reading them was not an easy task because, without fail, the reading triggered the symptoms of acute panic attack. Almost every page I read reminded me of the worst I'd been through. Just picking up such a book would give me severe physical symptoms of anxiety. It made me want to throw it away, crawl into a ball and wait for the pain to dissipate. Sometimes I did just that, taking time to recuperate. I knew I wasn't going to die and that those symptoms, painful as they were, were just the body's reaction to perceived but non-existent danger.

Eventually, my persistence would take over and I continued to battle through reading and learning, eventually to be victorious.

From books I learned that children who had to grow up fast, tending to their family, are likely to have panic attacks when they grow up. Usually it would be the oldest child in a family. There was a lot of information on the connection between perfectionism and anxiety, diet and anxiety, as well as other triggers and predispositions. I am extremely grateful that I liked research and learning, as it served me and empowered me.

Various Specialists

At the very beginning of this whole ordeal, the first symptom I had was tightness in my shoulders and neck. I thought it was logical to see a chiropractor. I experienced some relief after a few sessions, but not completely. In a few days, I felt tightness in my chest and some numbness down my left arm. When these symptoms persisted and even worsened I thought I'd better see a cardiologist, which I did. After numerous tests, I was assured my symptoms were not due to a major heart problem and was relieved. Doctors found some abnormality, but I was in no danger and didn't even need medication for the heart condition I had. It put me somewhat at ease, but I was still suffering a great deal. My anxiety was much more than nervousness in stressful situations and I sought qualified professionals with whom I was comfortable talking and whom I trusted. I believe in seeking second or third opinions and even changing healthcare providers if something didn't feel right. My health was my responsibility and even though I often felt totally out of control in my own body, I pushed through, looking for cure. Over time, I assembled a healing team of various specialists.

I was in the care of my family physician, seeing a psychologist and was evaluated by a psychiatrist for disability. I believe far too many people are living in denial, afraid to admit there is anything wrong with them, thus refusing to seek help. What if they go to see a doctor and get a diagnosis of a disturbing mental illness? In this information age, way too many people suffer for fear of the unknown. Admittedly, facing inner demons is scary; it is so much easier to do nothing, not forcing yourself to be brave and fight even if the possible outcome is wellbeing and happiness.

An old joke comes to mind about a guy drowning in a river. God sends him a boat, a raft and a log, but the man refuses help, waiting for His divine intervention. When this man finally drowned and went to heaven, he asked God why He did not rescue him. Then God answered: who do you think sent your way all those floating devices you so foolishly refused?! This can illustrate that when we look for healing, God sends doctors, other health care providers, medication, and psychologists to help us when needed.

Psychological Help

Though I was glad to be diagnosed early on, I was not ecstatic to learn that I had panic disorder, as I had not yet been free of the idea of stigma. I was clinging to the secondary diagnosis of mild heart condition, using it initially as the apparent cause of my hospitalization to family and friends.

I am so glad I didn't have to be admitted to a hospital for mental patients. I had a fleeting suicidal thought, which disappeared, thankfully, not to come back. Years ago, my close relative had to spend a few weeks at the psychiatric ward and I was told it was a horrible experience. It was a different country and different time, but even in beautiful California, being admitted to a mental institution is not something to brag about and nothing to look forward to. With mental disorders so prevalent now, the stigma becomes less and less. But at that time, I was burning with shame when I was not able to return to work, but greatly relieved to know that the only time I was admitted to a hospital was at the very beginning, when my heart had to be checked. I was also grateful that I could use a mild heart condition as my excuse for not returning to teaching. I was a total mess inside, yet for a while I concealed it in conversations, even with close friends, because I was painfully ashamed.

Many people turn to psychologists as a last resort, the same way they wait until the bitter end to seek specialists in other areas of life: finances, marriage, life choices etc. There are caring and highly educated people who specialize in all issues of relationship and mental health. This type of expense should be categorized as a necessity, similar to health, dental, house and auto maintenance.

As so many others with emotional and physical distress, I was not yet convinced I needed to see a psychologist, but was forced, due to absence from work. This turned out in my favor, so I'm glad I did it early on. The first psychologist lent me a book and CD with exercises for overcoming panic. I followed the recommendations as was prescribed. The only exercise I remember is drawing an imaginary circle on the floor around me to feel protected. At first it sounded bizarre, but I gave it a try. I was determined to try even the silly or flat out crazy. And if such advice was found in a book written by a distinguished Ph.D., it only strengthened my resolve to submit. Drawing those imaginary circles around me on the bathroom floor sounded almost pagan, but it did indeed give me a strange feeling of being sheltered and protected, and I know they were designed to represent the boundary of protection from the outside world. Later I read about using a hula-hoop to create a similar boundary. In any case, creating these circles was beneficial for someone who thought she was completely losing her mind. It was a temporary fix because I felt I was a total mess.

My first therapist was very nice, but specialized in family and marriage counseling. By the time of my last insurance-covered visit, I was nowhere near being well, so I looked up an anxiety specialist. With the help of my physician, I got a list of my insurance providers, narrowed it down to my preference of female specialists in the area and checked references. I chose a psychologist I thought best to address my needs and made my first appointment. I was prepared to see a few psychologists from my list to choose the one I was the most comfortable with—after all, during therapy sessions, I would bare my very soul and unearth many deeply hidden issues I told no one about. I was relieved that I felt comfortable with the very first anxiety specialist I saw. I stayed in therapy for almost a year and it was very helpful. During those sessions, long-repressed thoughts and experiences gushed from me as streams of cleansing water, verbalized for the first time. They trickled at first, then the floodgates opened and I wept, fully experiencing relief. In the past, when painful events happened, I didn't allow myself to properly grieve, shoving all the emotions deep inside, covering them with a veneer of "I don't give a damn" attitude. Obviously, that backfired. Talking to a mental care professional met a need to express my thoughts and emotions in confidence, but with the realization that I am not my thoughts and feelings, I only experience them, which was very helpful.

After a while, I was telling my therapist that I would like to find a life coach. I wanted to create sort of an action plan for my future and move forward faster. Though life coaching not her specialty, she helped me by providing what she was trained to do: listening as I spilled my emotions and pain, guiding me to open up and look for emotional patterns in my stories, bringing me to realization what in many instances was holding me back.

When I think I am sick with an ear infection, severe stomachache or flu, I go straight to the doctor's office, describe my symptoms and expect to be treated. Once properly diagnosed, anxiety, as well as depression and anger, are as treatable and curable as other diseases.

Unfortunately, I am addicted to instant gratification. If not all of us, definitely a majority of us want immediate healing. Unfortunately, healing takes time and there is no magic pill that could cure me completely and on the spot. There are drugs to make me feel better instantly (halleluiah!) by changing my biochemistry in a matter of minutes. The first few times I took it, the effect felt good. But I didn't want to get addicted to pills (or anything else). Also, the emotional numbness and fog made me avoid long-term medication, so I used them only as a last resort. I kept them in my purse and just knowing that I can take them was like a safety net, though this was not a long-term solution.

I respected my doctor's opinions but I wanted to fully participate in the healing process. It was my responsibility to choose the treatment that I was comfortable with. I turned to many health care providers, but I was also doing my homework.

By working with psychologists, I learned to ask myself deep questions and to discover motives for my fears, longings and other emotions. When I ponder a question for a while, I can come with an answer. It usually wells up inside and comes out with tears. I was wondering why on many occasions I was thinking about leaving my home church I was a member of for over a decade. The answer emerged and I felt very sad and emotional, I know... I was longing for stability and belonging for a very long time. Our little church in Malibu is a very nice place but it went through numerous transitions. People come and go. When I come in now I hardly see any familiar faces. I became an expert of asking the right questions to figure out roots of my internal conflicts. I can even help those close to me to figure out what really bothers them.

Desperate Need of Self-Care

Juggling a career, a household with its endless errands and chores at times leave me feel tired, unlovable and even resentful. Without taking care of myself, I am often unable to care for my beloved family and people close to me the way I truly want. Long gone are times when I tried to manipulate others to pity me; now I learn to delegate. When "my glass is empty," I can't share "living water" of my life with others. I need to take time to fill up. The best way to do it is to spend time in being still in God's presence. Reading the Scriptures, praying and listening in silence are necessary and refreshing to soul, mind and body. We need to allot uninterrupted time for this purpose without feeling guilty that we are not productive.

There are also days when I simply need to stay in my pajamas, watch old movies and eat comfort food. Then there are days when I can eat salads, go for a walk or work out and organize my drawers and closets. Both ways can help to refocus and recharge batteries. I want to mention that we need to be aware when problem avoidance and escapism lasts for months and we become reluctant, lazy or afraid to venture into the real world. So a plan should be developed to get out of this vicious circle of despondency, depression and lethargy. There is a way to live fully, moving forward in a healthy pace.

We all need to seek balance in our lives. Self-care is necessary, using simple antidotes: down-time with a magazine or a book, a silly comedy or a little sketch on YouTube, a walk or a run, face-to-face time with girlfriends, or just a phone chat.

When I am really pressed on time but I need this "girl time" I may have a cup of coffee with a girlfriend on Skype or Face Time, wearing my pajamas. Hooray for technology! Sometimes, when the pile-up of things to do gets too much and life seems to be spinning out of control, extreme self-care measures need to be scheduled and implemented, even if it seems there is no time. Women especially often feel guilty for not being productive or being selfish in taking care of themselves. Occasionally it'll take a drastic measure of scheduling a massage, a haircut or manicure, an adults-only dinner or a trip—all the good stuff. It does not have to be expensive; there are ways to barter goods and services with other women in my circle. Where there's a will, there's a way—proven!

The Art of Waiting and Resting

You may not expect a life coach to recommend waiting; after all, coaching is about taking action, completing tasks and beating procrastination. Sure, taking action is important, but there are times when we need to pause and compose ourselves before taking a leap. I learned the hard way the importance of rest, but I can be a slow learner, and my God, my teacher used whatever methods He saw fit. He Himself took a break after creating the world. That should've been a clue, but of course, I didn't learn from somebody else's example, silly me! God chose to take this time off and actually commanded us to have such a day of complete rest -- doing nothing for a day, on a weekly basis. Jesus, after preaching, healing and ministering, had to withdraw to have a time of reflection, prayer and solitude. I had to learn the importance of this practice, but not at once. I was anxious and frustrated, wondering why I was not able to shake off darkness that seemed to cling on and blind me. I wanted to move forward and find out what to do next. Last thing I wanted to do was to lay dormant and wait. But I had to hang on and reflect at first, learning patience from God's Creation. All kinds of analogies resurfaced to teach me.

A seed goes into the ground to die as a seed and to grow into a daisy, a head of cabbage or a mighty oak, but if you don't know what kind of seed you are planting, you will not know what to expect. From a tiny seed that you can barely see, a huge tree can eventually grow, given proper care and conditions. A caterpillar eats leaves, grows bigger and bigger, then it makes a cocoon around itself, where it undergoes metamorphosis, being totally transformed while hidden from view, to emerge in due time as a beautiful butterfly. We only have to wait and see. None of us know for sure how our lives will turn out, but those times come when we need to go into complete stillness, hidden from the eyes of others, to undergo complete transformation, and to emerge as an entirely new creation.

A time of solitude was, after all, necessary for my growth. But after a while, it felt like prison. I got very tired of being dormant. It took time for me to break through my "cocoon." Eventually I did spread my wings and found that I can fly. Another way to look at it is that I had to slowly emerge and grow from the darkness, as a vine trying to hold onto anything within reach for support, but inevitably growing stronger and taller, reaching for the sun.

Conclusion

On its own, your thoughts can drift randomly from one idea to another, it can go down memory lane, chase wild thoughts, or stir up bitter ideas or resentment and anger. Alternatively, your mind can dive into a sea of daydreaming and a world of fantasy, if care is not taken, your life can be controlled by such random thoughts such that every decision or action you take becomes unpredictable. Such intrusive thoughts you might experience during the day is evidence that most of the functions of the mind are likely beyond conscious control. In addition, our thoughts can feel so powerful and real and it can affect the way we perceive the outside world.

Take a moment to discard the assumption that your spontaneous thoughts are meaningless and totally harmless. In truth, such thoughts may be meaningless at that moment, they can be the product of past memory or emotion but in the present moment, they might not reflect reality.

Most of our thoughts are under the control of our subconscious mind and our subconscious mind will never grant us total control over our thoughts. However, you still have the capacity to control some of your thoughts. Also, you can change some of your habits and how you react to them to gain more control over your emotions.

As you went through this book, you have found a various selection of ideas and tools that can help you to declutter your mind so that you can mute all the negative voices in your head, reduce stress, and have more peace of mind.

Making conscious efforts to avoid overthinking is a rewarding course of action which will impact the quality of your life significantly. By spending less time going through intrusive, negative thoughts "in your mind" you will have more time to enjoy the present moment and every other moment.